T0234370

Women's Health in Interventional Radiology

Elizabeth Ann Ignacio • Anthony C. Venbrux
(Editors)

Women's Health in Interventional Radiology

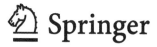 Springer

Editors

Elizabeth Ann Ignacio
The George Washington University
Medical Center
Department of Radiology
Division of Interventional Radiology
900 23rd St NW
Washington, DC 20037
USA

Anthony C. Venbrux
The George Washington University
Medical Center
Department of Radiology
Division of Interventional Radiology
900 23rd St NW
Washington, DC 20037
USA

ISBN 978-1-4419-5875-4   e-ISBN 978-1-4419-5876-1
DOI 10.1007/978-1-4419-5876-1
Springer New York Dordrecht Heidelberg London

Library of Congress Control Number: 2011939211

Printed on acid-free paper

Springer is part of Springer Science+Business Media (www.springer.com)

*For my family, my lovely husband, Charles,
and especially my mother, Eleodora – thank
you so much for your endless love
and support.*

EAI

*To Michael Heinl, who believes in me.
To all those whom I have had the privilege
of teaching.
To our patients, who have taught
us so much about life.*

ACV

Foreword

I am honored to have been asked to contribute a few words regarding this first edition of *Women's Health in Interventional Radiology*. Having spent much of my professional energy for the past decade in interventional practice in Women's Health, I am pleased that a comprehensive guide to the field is now available, and reviewing it has been a pleasure.

What struck me first about this text is the breadth of topics that are addressed. It focuses not just on interventions in the female reproductive tract, but on all the major interventions that have a major impact on Women's Health. The inclusion of lower extremity venous insufficiency and osteoporotic spinal compression fractures is in recognition of the disproportionate impact that these pathologies have on women and their quality of life. In turn, women are the primary beneficiaries of recent advances in interventional therapies for those conditions. As a result, this book provides the means for those already practicing in women's intervention to increase their knowledge in those procedures in which they are already active and the opportunity to broaden their scope of care to new procedures. This book is ideal for those who would like to dedicate themselves to high quality of Women's Health at all stages of life.

Dr. Venbrux and Dr. Ignacio have long been active in the field of women's interventions, and they have assembled a similarly dedicated group of authors. Their commitment to excellence comes through on every page. I congratulate them on an outstanding new contribution to our field, one that I hope will advance our knowledge but also our commitment to ensuring the best case outcome for those we are privileged to treat.

Washington, DC, USA   James B. Spies, M.D., MPH

Preface

In the last 20 years, national and international interest has become increasingly focused on Women's Health. Throughout the world, this important health care discipline has traditionally been underserved and specific conditions undertreated. The National Women Health Network (1975), the Women's Health Initiative of the National Institutes of Health (1991), and the Global Alliance for Women's Health of the United Nations (1994) are a few examples of the many comprehensive efforts to increase education, advocacy, research, and resources for Women's Health issues.

Interventional Radiology, a medical field known for its creativity and innovation in procedural patient care, continues to deliver inventive and resourceful methods for caring for women in all stages of life. In the average Interventional Radiology practice, Women's Health may represent a significant component branch of the practice. Furthermore, the contemporary Interventional Radiologist, assuming more clinical responsibility than his or her predecessors, now has office hours, admissions, and follow-up management protocols that are standard and an integral part of daily patient care operations. As we face a challenging and demanding field with a rapidly expanding body of scientific knowledge, particularly in the area of Women's Health, it is important to provide texts that present a clear, concise, and timely overview of the subject matter.

This book will highlight those Interventional Radiology procedures most pertinent to Women's Health. The authors have labored to cover the sections completely, providing a detailed discussion of pathophysiology, techniques, clinical notes, and a broad review of the literature. Additionally, the authors have distilled information into a concise format so that the actual book has portability.

We hope this book can be a working text, on hand for the Interventional Radiologist in the office or as he or she makes rounds in the hospital. We trust that our readers will find this manual of practical assistance in the work-up, procedural treatment, and management of patients. If this book meets the educational goals of the reader, then the time, energy, and effort expended in its preparation will be justified.

We wish to express our gratitude to our talented and experienced colleagues who contributed to this book. They are a constant source of inspiration and motivation, and we are appreciative of their dedication and concerted efforts.

Elizabeth Ann Ignacio, M.D.
Anthony C. Venbrux, M.D.

Disclaimer

There are many commercial products that are specifically listed in each of the chapters of this book. The editors and contributors have given their personal and anecdotal description of specific product use in order to be helpful. However, with only one exception (Wayne Olan, M.D.), the editors and authors are not affiliated with or have financial interest in the products mentioned.

Further, absolutely none of the editors and authors received any financial incentive to discuss any of the specific products mentioned in this book.

Contents

Contributors

Farhang Adabi, RTR
Department of Radiology,
Division of Interventional Radiology,
The George Washington University
Medical Center, Washington,
DC, USA

Yousaf Awan, M.D.
Department of Radiology,
University of Maryland Medical Center,
Baltimore, MD, USA

Chad Baarson, DO
Department of Radiology,
National Capitol Consortium,
Bethesda, MD, USA

Jozef M. Brozyna, B.S., B.A.
West Virginia School of Osteopathic
Medicine, Lewisburg, WV, USA

Albert K. Chun, M.D.
Department of Radiology,
Division of Interventional Radiology,
The George Washington University
Medical Center, Washington, DC, USA

Sameul Hanif, M.D.
The George Washington University
Medical Center, Washington, DC, USA

Amy P. Harper, MSN, ACNP-BC
Division of Radiology, Division of
Interventional Radiology,
The George Washington University
Medical Center, Washington, DC, USA

Taara Sultaana Hassan, M.D.
The George Washington University School
of Medicine, Washington, DC, USA

Aaron Himchak, M.D.
Department of Radiology Morristown
Medical Center, Morristown, NJ, USA

Lena Hover, RTR
Department of Radiology,
Division of Interventional Radiology,
The George Washington University
Medical Center, Washington, DC, USA

Elizabeth Ann Ignacio, M.D.
Department of Radiology, Division of
Interventional Radiology,
The George Washington University
Medical Center, Washington, DC, USA

**Emily Timmreck Jackson, MSN,
ACNP-BC**
Department of Radiology,
Division of Interventional Radiology,
The George Washington University
Medical Center, Washington, DC, USA

Jay Karajgikar, B.A.
Department of Radiology, The George
Washington University Medical Center,
Washington, DC, USA

Jason B. Katzen, M.D.
Department of Radiology,
The George Washington University
Medical Center, Washington, DC, USA

Nadia J. Khati, M.D.
Department of Radiology,
Division of Body Imaging,
The George Washington University
Medical Center, Washington,
DC, USA

Sarah LaFond, M.D.
The George Washington University School
of Medicine, Washington, DC, USA

John C. Lipman, M.D., FSIR
Interventional Radiology,
Atlanta Interventional Institute,
Emory Adventist Hospital,
Atlanta, GA, USA

Wayne J. Olan, M.D.
Department of Neurosurgery,
Division of Interventional Radiology,
The George Washington University
Medical Center, Washington, DC, USA

Denis Primakov, M.D.
Department of Radiology,
National Naval Medical Center,
Bethesda, MD, USA

Shawn N. Sarin, M.D.
Department of Radiology, Division of
Interventional Radiology,
The George Washington University
Medical Center, Washington, DC, USA

Giriraj K. Sharma, M.D., M.S.
Department of Radiology,
The George Washington University
Medical Center, Washington, DC, USA

Prasanna Vasudevan, M.D., B.S.
Department of Radiology,
The George Washington University
Medical Center, Washington, DC, USA

Anthony C. Venbrux, M.D.
Department of Radiology,
Division of Interventional Radiology,
The George Washington University
Medical Center, Washington, DC, USA

Ajay D. Wadgaonkar, M.D.
The Russel H. Morgan Department of
Radiology and Radiological Science,
The Johns Hopkins Hospital,
Baltimore, MD, USA

Part I

Pelvic Vascular Interventions

Uterine Artery Embolization

1

Shawn N. Sarin, Chad Baarson, Sameul Hanif,
Yousaf Awan, and Anthony C. Venbrux

Introduction

Uterine artery embolization has become a significant interventional procedure that is performed electively to treat symptoms related to symptomatic uterine leiomyoma. This chapter will deal with elective workup and management of uterine leiomyoma.

The traditional treatment for symptomatic leiomyomata has primarily consisted of surgery, either hysterectomy or myomectomy (surgical removal of leiomyomata without hysterectomy). Hysterectomy has been considered the definitive treatment for leiomyomata because there is no chance of post-procedure recurrence. However, there are disadvantages of hysterectomy, including an estimated overall complication rate of 17–23% regardless of approach (abdominal, transvaginal, or laparoscopic) [1]. Hysterectomy is not appropriate for women who wish to preserve fertility. Myomectomy allows for women to retain their uterus, but there is a chance that an emergent hysterectomy may need to be performed due to excessive intraoperative bleeding. Also, symptoms due to uterine fibroids often recur in patients who have undergone myomectomy due to continued growth of remaining leiomyomata. In one study, the cumulative incidence of a repeat surgery due to fibroid recurrence was 23.5% at 5 years and 30% at 7 years [2]. Therefore, despite the fact that myomectomy allows for uterine retention, there is a significant risk of the need for additional surgery.

Uterine Artery Embolization (UAE) is a less invasive alternative to treating symptomatic uterine fibroids that preserves the uterus. In 1997, UAE was utilized in the United States for the first time in treating symptomatic uterine fibroids. This technique was described by Goodwin et al. [3]. UAE requires transcatheter embolization of the uterine arteries and devascularizes the leiomyomata. This is accomplished by delivering particulate emboli, such as polyvinyl alcohol particles or microspheres, into both uterine arteries. This markedly decreases blood flow at the arteriolar level. As a result, an irreversible ischemic injury to the fibroid is produced while preserving uterine function in the majority of cases.

S.N. Sarin (✉)
Department of Radiology, Division of Interventional Radiology,
The George Washington University Medical Center, Washington, DC, USA
e-mail: ssarin@gwu.edu

E.A. Ignacio and A.C. Venbrux (eds.), *Women's Health in Interventional Radiology*,
DOI 10.1007/978-1-4419-5876-1_1, © Springer Science+Business Media, LLC 2012

UAE has become increasingly popular and is an effective method in treating symptomatic uterine fibroids. The Society of Interventional Radiology (SIR) reports that 13,000–14,000 UAE procedures have been performed annually in the USA since 2004. The American College of Obstetricians and Gynecologists (ACOG) issued a statement on UAE saying that its treatment of symptomatic fibroids, when performed by experienced physicians, appears to provide good short-term relief among appropriate candidates, with low complication rates [4]. Due to lack of long-term data (10 years), UAE is currently not recommended for women who intend to become pregnant. However, there have been reported cases in which women have become pregnant after undergoing UAE, and therefore this procedure does not preclude subsequent pregnancy.

Advantages of UAE in comparison to hysterectomy and myomectomy are substantial and include similar efficacy with less serious complications, retention of the uterus, overnight or outpatient hospital stay, more rapid recovery time, and treatment for patients who are not candidates for surgery. Although long-term data are not yet available, initial trials have documented that regrowth of embolized fibroids is rare.

Pathophysiology

The uterus is made up of two major components: the endometrium and myometrium. The myometrium is the site of uterine fibroids. The endometrium normally lines the internal cavity of the uterus and is composed of glands that are embedded in a cellular stroma. The endometrium is the part of the uterus that undergoes morphologic changes during the menstrual cycle in response to hormones produced by the ovaries. Leiomyomata develop in the myometrium portion of the uterus, which is composed of tightly interwoven bundles of smooth muscle that form the wall of the uterus. These leiomyomata derive their main blood supply almost exclusively from the uterine arteries [5].

Uterine fibroids are benign smooth muscle neoplasms originating in the myometrium that may occur singly, but most often are multiple. These tumors are the most common benign gynecological neoplasm in women of reproductive age. The exact etiology of leiomyomata is not known. There are several factors that play a key role in the development of fibroids. Evidence suggests that estrogen and estrogen receptors are vital to the pathogenesis of fibroids. Uterine leiomyomata tend to occur during the reproductive period, a time when hormonal influences (including estrogen) are at a peak. Also, these fibroids initially become apparent after menarche, enlarge during pregnancy, and regress after menopause, which further supports the concept that hormones play a key part in fibroid development. Some studies comparing leiomyomata to normal myometrium have shown that leiomyomata have an abnormal gene expression that maintains a high level of sensitivity to estrogen during the estrogen-dominated proliferative phase of the menstrual cycle. Additionally, when comparing cultured myometrial cells with cultured cells from leiomyomata in the same patient, there is a higher response to estrogen in the latter group. Furthermore, semiquantitative immunohistochemical demonstration of estrogen and progesterone receptors correlates with the growth rate of the fibroids [6].

In addition to the effect of estrogen on the pathogenesis of uterine fibroids, genetic and chromosomal abnormalities seem to play a role [6, 7]. Although the majority of leiomyomata have normal karyotypes, up to 40% have a simple chromosomal abnormality.

Morphologically, leiomyomata have distinct features macroscopically and microscopically. On gross examination, uterine fibroids are sharply circumscribed, round, discrete, firm, gray-white tumors that may vary in size from being barely visible nodules to very large tumors. Generally, they are located within the corpus of the uterus; however, they may involve the uterine ligaments, lower uterine segment, or even the cervix, which is outside the uterus. Although these tumors are in the myometrium (intramural), they may be situated very close to the endometrium (submucosal) or close to the serosa (subserosal). Due to the varied location of these fibroids within the myometrium, they may protrude into the uterine cavity or into the peritoneum. Submucosal fibroids are the ones that typically lead to intermenstrual bleeding since the mucosal surface may atrophy or erode as it they protrude into the uterine cavity. Regardless of their size and location, uterine leiomyomata have the characteristic whorled pattern of smooth muscle bundles on cut section, which makes them easily identifiable on gross examination. Furthermore, large fibroids may develop areas of yellow-brown to red softening, known as red degeneration.

Microscopically, leiomyomata consist of whorled bundles of smooth muscle cells similar in appearance to normal myometrium. Although leiomyomata are neoplasms of smooth muscle cells, mitotic figures are scarce, which is one of the main criteria that are used to distinguish fibroids from leiomyosarcomas (malignant neoplasms).

There are several benign variants of leiomyomata including symplastic tumor, benign metastasizing leiomyoma, and disseminated peritoneal leiomyomatosis. Symplastic tumors are atypical or bizarre neoplasms with nuclear atypia, giant cells, and cellular leiomyomata. Benign metastasizing leiomyomata consist of a uterine tumor that extends into vessels and migrates to other sites such as the lung. Disseminated peritoneal leiomyomatosis presents as multiple small nodules on the peritoneum. Even though these last two variants have unusual characteristics and show signs of invasion, they are still considered benign.

Clinical Manifestations

A uterine fibroid or leiomyoma is a benign tumor that originates from the myometrium (smooth muscle layer) of the uterus, and it is the most common benign tumor of females. Patients typically present in the mid to late reproductive years, and the true prevalence of leiomyomata is underestimated. One study showed that, in a random sampling of women aged 35–49 who were screened by self-report, medical record review, and sonography, Caucasian women had an incidence of 40% by age 35, which increased to about 70% by age 50. In that same study, African-American women had an incidence of 60% by age 35 and as high as 80% by age 50 [8].

Uterine fibroids are noncancerous tumors that are generally asymptomatic and usually do not require treatment. The most common symptoms of uterine fibroid problems are heavy menstrual bleeding and pelvic pain. Uterine leiomyomata can sometimes enlarge and cause menorrhagia, dyspareunia, urinary urgency and frequency, constipation, or hydronephrosis due to compression of the ureters. Once any of these symptoms begin to interfere with daily life and activities, then treatment for leiomyomata is indicated.

Uterine leiomyomata do have some relationship with patient infertility, but it is still controversial what exact mechanical or physiologic problems their presence may effect in the reproductive tract of the infertile patient. Myomas may lead to problems with conception, especially if they are near the fallopian tubes, partially or completely obstructing the passage of the egg and sperm for fertilization. Submucosal fibroids that bulge into the uterine cavity may possibly cause early miscarriage [9]. Studies investigating the treatment of submucosal fibroids in patients with subfertility have shown increased assisted pregnancy rates following directed therapy. While some investigators have hypothesized that the uterine lining at the fibroid site can be thinned with a decreased blood supply for implantation and growth of the developing embryo, others argue that there is no difference in the endometrium overlying these fibroids compared to that overlying other areas of the uterus [10]. Despite these questions, in patients with otherwise unexplained infertility, fibroids that are submucosal, larger than 5 cm, or distort the uterine cavity are often treated as the possible cause.

Anatomy

Pelvic Arterial Anatomy

Understanding the pelvic vascular anatomy as well as anatomic variants is fundamental to safe and effective embolization. Care should be taken to identify the branches of the internal iliac artery to avoid non-target embolization. Knowledge of anatomic variants also is important to ensure safety of the procedure.

The *internal iliac artery* supplies the walls and viscera of the pelvis as well as the buttock and medial side of the thigh [11] (Fig. 1.1). It arises at the junction of the common and external iliac arteries at approximately the lumbosacral junction, passes inferiorly, at approximately the level of the superior portion of the greater sciatic foramen, and bifurcates into an anterior trunk and a posterior trunk in 57–77% of the population [5]. The internal iliac artery demonstrates 90% bilateral symmetry of its branching patterns [5]. The anterior trunk branches into three vesical arteries (superior, middle, and inferior), the middle hemorrhoidal artery, obturator artery, internal pudendal artery, inferior gluteal artery, and the uterine and vaginal arteries. The posterior trunk gives off the superior gluteal artery, iliolumbar artery, and the lateral sacral artery.

The *uterine artery* is a branch of the anterior division of the internal iliac artery. This artery supplies the ureter, uterus, vagina, round ligament of the uterus, fallopian tube, and part of the ovary. There are four different variants of the uterine artery. Type I (45%) arises from the first branch of the inferior gluteal artery; Type II (6%) arises from the second or third branch of the inferior gluteal artery; Type III (15–43%) is defined as a trifurcation with the origins of the inferior gluteal artery, superior gluteal artery, and uterine arteries; Type IV (6%) with the uterine artery origin arising proximal to the bifurcation of the anterior and posterior divisions [5, 11, 84]. It may be the first or the second branch from the inferior gluteal artery in 51% of patients [5, 12]. Greater than 90% of patients demonstrate bilateral symmetry of the branching pattern of the internal iliac arteries [5]. If the internal

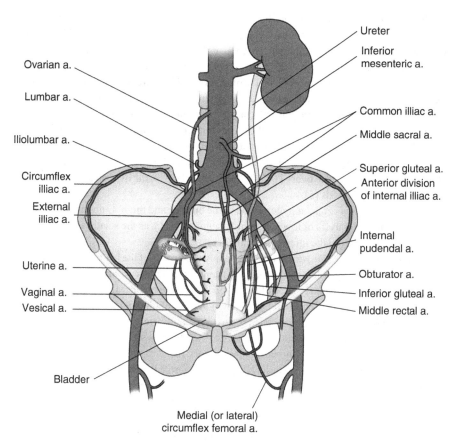

Ovarian a.

Lumbar a.

Iliolumbar a.

Circumflex
  illiac a.

External
  illiac a.

Uterine a.

Vaginal a.

Vesical a.

Bladder

Ureter

Inferior
mesenteric a.

Common illiac a.

Middle sacral a.

Superior gluteal a.
Anterior division
of internal illiac a.

Internal
pudendal a.

Obturator a.

Inferior gluteal a.

Middle rectal a.

Medial (or lateral)
circumflex femoral a.

Fig. 1.1 Pelvic arterial anatomy

iliac artery is divided into two main trunks, the best projection to identify the origin of the uterine artery is the contralateral anterior oblique with 20–30° of inclination [1].

The uterine artery demonstrates a "U" shape with a descending segment that runs medial on the levator ani and toward the cervix. The uterine artery then crosses transversely above and in front of the ureter, to reach the side wall of the uterus. Here, the uterine artery ascends in a tortuous manner between two layers of the broad ligament to the uterine margin. The uterine artery can then deviate laterally toward the ovary, eventually anastomosing with the ovarian artery.

The uterine artery has several branches. First, there is the cervicovaginal artery, which arises from the transverse segment. This artery should be spared during embolization. Non-target embolization of the cervicovaginal artery has been associated with reported complications such as labial necrosis [12]. Second, there are the intramural (arcuate) arteries, which course through the outer third of the myometrium [5]. The uterine artery may be replaced by small arterial branches or may be absent. If so, it is often replaced by the ipsilateral ovarian artery.

The *ovarian artery* arises from abdominal aorta just inferior to the renal arteries in 80–90% cases [5]. It demonstrates a characteristic corkscrew appearance. The ovarian artery can arise from the renal, lumbar, adrenal, or iliac artery [5]. The ovaries are perfused by either the ovarian arteries in 40% of cases, both the uterine and ovarian arteries in 56% of cases, or the uterine arteries alone in 4% of cases [5]. There are three defined patterns of anastomosis of the ovarian–uterine arteries. Types Ia and Ib define the ovarian artery as the primary source of blood to the fibroid via the anastomotic connection with the uterine artery. Ia (13.2%) defines flow toward the uterus without retrograde flow to the ovary, and Ib (8.6%) defines flow toward the uterus with reflux into the ovarian artery. Type II (3.9%) is defined as direct supply of blood to the fibroid tumors. Type III (6.6%) defines flow in the uterine artery toward the ovary [11, 12]. In 5–10% of cases, the ovarian arteries provide flow to the uterine fibroids [5].

The *inferior gluteal artery* supplies blood to the buttock and thigh. Embolization of this artery may lead to paralysis of lower extremity segments [11], as the sciatic artery supplying the nerve arises from the inferior gluteal artery.

The *superior and inferior vesical arteries* supply the fundus of the bladder and the lower ureter. These arteries may arise as a common trunk with the uterine artery. The vesicular branches supply approximately 80% of the blood flow to the bladder [5]. To avoid bladder necrosis, special consideration should be given to avoid embolization of these vessels.

The *round ligament artery* arises from the external iliac artery or from inferior epigastric artery. It plays a minor role in uterine vascular supply. Persistent bleeding after hysterectomy may be related to round ligament artery injury [5].

It is essential to preserve the posterior trunk of the internal iliac artery as embolization of this artery may lead to lower extremity complications (e.g., buttock and hip claudication).

The *iliolumbar artery* divides into the lumbar and iliac branches. The lumbar branch anastomoses with the fourth lumbar artery and supplies blood to the ventral rami of L5, S1, and S2. The iliac branch has anastomoses with the superior gluteal, circumflex iliac, and the lateral circumflex femoral arteries [11].

The *superior gluteal artery* is the largest branch off of the posterior trunk supplying the gluteus maximus muscle with multiple anastomotic connections.

Imaging

Conventional radiographs have a limited role in the diagnosis of uterine fibroids because only heavily calcified fibroids are depicted. Extreme enlargement of the uterus resulting from fibroids may be seen as a nonspecific soft-tissue mass of the pelvis that possibly displaces loops of bowel (Fig. 1.2a).

CT scanning also has a limited role in the diagnosis of uterine fibroids (Fig. 1.2b). On CT, fibroids are usually indistinguishable from normal myometrium unless they are calcified or necrotic. Calcifications are typically more visible on CT scans than on conventional radiographs because of the superior contrast differentiation.

Air may be seen on CT scans in the fibroid following UAE. Acutely, this may be air that is introduced during the embolization procedure. Later, it may represent air/gas filling potential spaces left by tissue infarction/desiccation. This may be seen on CT as early as

Fig. 1.2 (**a**) Abdomen AP image shows a paucity of gas in the right and mid-abdomen. Findings suggest a mass but are nonspecific. (**b**) Axial CT scan abdomen of same patient. Large fibroid uterus

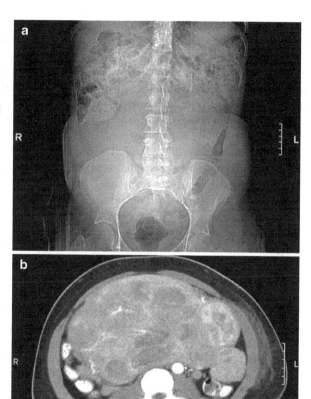

1 month post procedure [13]. Rarely does air/gas in the fibroid represent infection. History, physical findings, and laboratory findings must be correlated to exclude infection.

The vast majority of patients with symptoms suspicious for uterine fibroids are initially worked up with transabdominal and or transvaginal pelvic ultrasound (US). US has been used to assess the uterus and pelvic structures prior to and following UAE. Prior to embolization, US can reveal or exclude embolization contraindications such as pelvic masses (malignancy), endometrosis, adenomyosis, pregnancy, and pedunculated fibroids. Following UAE, US can be used to monitor post-procedure fibroid response or identify any complications (fibroid expulsion, sloughing, endometritis, and abscess) [14].

Fibroids are well-defined masses within the uterus. Dystrophic calcification within the fibroid may be present and create significant shadowing on ultrasound that can obscure evaluation of the uterus. Additionally, calcification on a preprocedure US can indicate the presence of involuted fibroids, which are unlikely to respond to UAE. There may be focal or global uterine enlargement. Depending on the location of the fibroid, there may be distortion of the endometrial echo complex. The uterine contour may be smooth or lobulated – related to subserosal fibroids. Submucosal fibroids may cause disruption or distortion of the endometrial lining [15, 16]. Standard US can generally define the characteristics, number, volume, and location of fibroids [17].

Sonohysterography is an important adjunct to transvaginal US in differentiating submucosal fibroids from endometrial polyps [15, 16]. This is clinically relevant since it is usually the submucosal leiomyoma that is responsible for abnormal uterine bleeding.

Uterine fibroid volumes are determined with a formula that uses the dimensions in the Anterior-Posterior (AP), Transverse, Craniocaudal (CC) planes multiplied by the correction factor 0.523 assuming an ellipsoid shape [18]. For example: $AP \times Transverse \times CC \times 0.5234$.

If multiple fibroids are present, the volumes of the codominant fibroids are measured, along with overall uterine volume. This can be monitored over time [19, 20].

Doppler evaluation or contrast enhanced ultrasound of fibroids is not routinely performed.

Adenomyosis, the presence of functioning endometrium within the myometrium, can be detected with ultrasound but it is not as sensitive or specific. However, US can differentiate fibroids from adenomyosis [21, 22]. The US appearance of adenomyosis includes myometrial cysts, ill-defined areas of myometrial echotexture, and a globular or enlarged uterus [23, 24]. UAE for symptomatic adenomyosis is controversial.

Endometriosis is a common disorder that may manifest with symptoms similar to those of symptomatic fibroids. These symptoms include bloating, pelvic pain, dyspareunia, rectal discomfort, and heavy menstrual periods. Endometriosis is poorly evaluated with ultrasound. Transvaginal US can identify ovarian endometriomas but is insensitive in identifying peritoneal implants [25]. Endometriomas appear as focal complex adnexal masses that may be unilocular or multilocular with diffuse low-level internal echoes.

Doppler flow evaluation of the uterine artery may have a role in evaluating patients for UAE. McLucas et al. [26] showed that Doppler flow US showed initial peak systolic velocity (PSV) correlated positively with size and shrinkage of myomas and overall uterine volume. A high pre-embolization PSV (>64 cm/s) was suggested as a predictor of UAE failure. Postembolization PSV did not show value in predicting clinical outcome [26].

Fibroids have a varied and complex US appearance prior to and following embolization, though some authors have reported that fibroids postembolization decrease in echogenicity [27].

Six to 12 months following embolization, US may reveal a hyperechoic rim representing peripheral calcification around an increasingly hypoechoic fibroid. This has been called the so-called "fetal head sign" [28]. The peripheral location of calcification following embolization differs from dystrophic calcification that is typically more central within the fibroid.

Occasionally, embolic particles may be seen within the uterine arteries following embolization. Color Doppler US usually shows a decrease in flow to the fibroids after embolization. Disappearance of intrafibroid vascularity is common, whereas flow in the perifibroid vessels can persist [29]. No correlation between embolization response and preprocedure color flow US appearance has been documented [27].

MR imaging is considered the most accurate imaging technique for detection and localization of leiomyomata [20, 30]. It can differentiate tissue planes between these benign tumors and has been shown to be more accurate than US [31]. Additionally, ultrasound has a limited field of view, preventing complete evaluation of an enlarged, fibroid uterus. This

Fig. 1.3 (**a, b**) Large pedunculated fibroid uterus rising out of true pelvis into abdomen. Previous attempted US (not shown) could not show entire uterus in the field of view

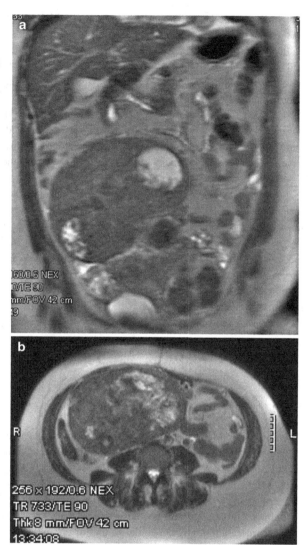

is not an issue with MR imaging [32] (Fig. 1.3a, b). MR imaging can differentiate uterine zonal anatomy, which allows accurate classification of submucosal, intramural, or subserosal fibroids [30]. MR has been shown to be more accurate than US or hysterosalpingography for determining the presence and location of fibroids in infertile women [31].

Viable (nondegenerated) leiomyomata on T2-weighted MR images are typically well-defined masses of homogeneously decreased signal intensity compared with that of the outer myometrium [30]. Pathologically, nondegenerated fibroids are composed of whorls of uniform smooth muscle cells with various amounts of intervening collagen [33]. Cellular leiomyomata, a benign leiomyoma variant, are composed of compact smooth muscle cells with little or no collagen. These can have relatively higher signal intensity on T2-weighted images and demonstrate enhancement on intravenous contrast-enhanced studies [34].

In contrast, degenerated leiomyomata have variable appearances on T2-weighted images and contrast-enhanced studies [35]. Leiomyomata with hyaline or calcific degeneration have low signal intensity on T2-weighted images, an appearance similar to that of standard leiomyomata. Leiomyomata with cystic degeneration show high signal intensity on T2-weighted images, and the cystic areas do not enhance. Leiomyomata with myxoid degeneration show very high signal intensity on T2-weighted images and enhance minimally on contrast-enhanced images. Necrotic leiomyomata that have not yet liquefied will have variable signal intensity on T1-weighted images and low signal intensity on T2-weighted images.

Leiomyomata with red degeneration may exhibit an unusual signal intensity pattern at MR imaging: peripheral or diffuse high signal intensity on T1-weighted images and variable signal intensity with or without a low signal intensity rim on T2-weighted images [36]. The high signal intensity on T1-weighted images is likely secondary to the proteinaceous content of the blood or the T1 shortening effects of methemoglobin [37]. When high signal intensity is isolated to the rim of the leiomyoma, it has been hypothesized that blood products are confined to thrombosed vessels that surround the tumor [36]. Some leiomyomata have a high-signal rim on T2-weighted images, which represents a pseudocapsule of dilated lymphatic vessels, dilated veins, or edema [38].

Differential Diagnosis on MR Imaging

Adenomyosis

As mentioned previously, adenomyosis is characterized pathologically by the presence of ectopic endometrial glands and stroma within the myometrium. This is associated with reactive hypertrophy of the surrounding myometrial smooth muscle [39]. Adenomyosis likely results from direct invasion of the myometrium by basal endometrium, though the cause of these phenomena is not well understood. Adenomyosis is most commonly a diffuse abnormality but may also occur as a focal mass, known as an adenomyoma [39]. The clinical presentation may be similar to that of uterine leiomyomata (dysmenorrhea and menorrahagia). On MR imaging, the diffuse form of adenomyosis appears as a thickened junctional zone (inner myometrium) on T2-weighted images [40, 41]. Although various normal ranges have been suggested, a junctional zone of 12 mm or thicker is highly suggestive of adenomyosis [42]. The low signal intensity of adenomyosis is due to the reactive, dense smooth muscle hypertrophy that surrounds the imbedded endometrial glands [43]. Small foci of high signal intensity of T2-weighted images represent the endometrial glands. Some of these ectopic foci of endometrium also have high signal intensity on T1-weighted images, a finding that corresponds to hemorrhage [43]. In its focal form, adenomyosis appears as an ill-defined area of low signal intensity within the myometrium on T2-weighted images [43], whereas leiomyomata often appear as well-circumscribed masses. As mentioned earlier, the role of UAE for treatment of symptomatic adenomyosis is unclear. Clinical studies are ongoing.

Solid Adnexal Mass

MR imaging allows differentiation of pedunculated leiomyomata from other types of adnexal masses. If there is continuity of an adnexal mass with the adjacent myometrium, then the diagnosis of leiomyoma can be established [44]. MR imaging has the ability to evaluate normal ovaries, even in the presence of an enlarged, myomatous uterus. This can help to determine the origin of pelvic masses by excluding a diagnosis of ovarian neoplasm [32]. Ovarian fibromas [45] and Brenner tumors [46] are benign masses that have a large fibrous component and can have signal characteristics similar to pedunculated leiomyoma. MR can show fibromas and Brenner tumors surrounded by ovarian stroma and follicles, thus establishing the ovarian origin of these tumors. Differentiation between uterine and ovarian processes is important in pregnant patients, since the confident diagnosis of a uterine leiomyoma may eliminate the need for surgery during pregnancy [47].

Focal Myometrial Contraction

Uterine contractions can simulate leiomyomata or focal adenomyosis on MR imaging. They can appear as a myometrial mass of low T2 signal. Because contractions are transient, resolution of the mass on follow-up imaging can help aid in establishing its diagnosis [48, 49].

Uterine Leiomyosarcoma

Sarcomatous degeneration of benign leiomyomata is a well-known process, though sarcomas can arise independently from the smooth muscle cells of the myometrium. It has been suggested that an irregular margin of a uterine leiomyoma at MR imaging is suggestive of sarcomatous transformation [50]. The specificity of this finding is not currently known. Additionally, the ability of MR imaging to allow differentiation of cellular or degenerated leiomyoma from leiomyosarcoma of the uterus has not been assessed. The diagnosis of leiomyosarcoma is often first established on pathology after surgical resection of a presumed benign uterine mass [51, 52].

Patient Encounter

Indications

UAE requires that the Interventional Radiologist assume an active clinical role in the diagnosis and management of patients with symptomatic leiomyomata. The Society of Interventional Radiology (SIR) Task Force on Uterine Artery Embolization recommends that embolization be offered only to patients with symptomatic uterine leiomyomata [53]. Patients who are reasonable candidates for UAE treatment may have symptoms of heavy menstrual bleeding, pelvic pain, or bulk symptoms from local compression of the bladder and the rectum.

Contraindications

Pregnancy is an absolute contraindication to UAE. Therefore, this should be excluded with a pregnancy test prior to the procedure.

Active infection is also a contraindication for embolization of any organ including the uterus because of the risk of abscess formation and infectious complications.

UAE for leiomyomata would also be contraindicated when leiomyosarcoma or other gynecologic malignancy is suspected unless the procedure is being performed for palliation or prior to resection.

Relative contraindications include an immunocompromised state, previous pelvic irradiation or surgery, chronic endometritis, a partially treated pelvic infection, or a large hydrosalpinx (especially in a patient with a history of sexually transmitted disease), all of which may predispose to infection after UAE.

Another relative contraindication to UAE is the desire to maintain childbearing potential, as preservation of fertility cannot be assured based on the current literature. Uncomplicated pregnancies and normal deliveries have been reported after UAE [54, 55], so this procedure may still be the preferred option for women who are not candidates for or who refuse myomectomy. At this time, there is insufficient information to predict the percentage of women who will be able to become pregnant after UAE. It is very likely that the chance of pregnancy will depend on the extent of the fibroids. Those patients with very extensive fibroids are probably less likely to become pregnant whether they have UAE, myomectomy, or even if they have no therapy at all. It should be noted, however, that a randomized controlled trial comparing UAE and myomectomy found superior reproductive outcomes after myomectomy in the first 2 years of follow-up [56].

Two recently published reviews of the literature conclude that myomectomy remains the standard of care for preserving fertility because of the increased risks of spontaneous abortion, preterm delivery, and abnormal placentation after UAE [57, 58]. It is unclear whether these increased risks are due to the presence of fibroids per se, the embolization, or a combination of the two. However, both studies also state that UAE should still be considered in patients who are not good candidates for myomectomy and in patients who refuse surgical management.

Concurrent use of a gonadotropin-releasing hormone agonist (Lupron®, leuprolide acetate, Abbott Laboratories, Abbott Park, Illinois) may impact on the technical success of the UAE procedure. As it works by attenuating the vascularity of the fibroid uterus, it can produce diffuse vasospasm during the embolization procedure. Some centers recommend that gonadotropin-releasing hormone agonists be stopped 6–8 weeks prior to UAE.

The size and location of the leiomyomata should also be considered. Enlargement of the uterus to greater than the equivalent of 20–24 weeks gestation may make adequate embolization difficult to accomplish. A subserosal leiomyoma that is attached by a narrow stalk (attachment point <50% of the diameter) can be at risk for detachment from the uterus, a situation that may result in aseptic peritonitis, and necessitate surgical intervention. A large submucosal leiomyoma (>10 cm in diameter) may present an increased risk for infection or prolonged discharge following embolization. The greater the ratio between the endometrial interface and diameter of a submucosal leiomyoma, the more likely that leiomyoma is to migrate into the endometrial cavity after UAE [59].

Other relative contraindications, similar to any interventional procedure, would include coagulopathy, severe contrast allergy, and renal impairment. Some of these problems may be treated prior to the procedure to reduce risk of adverse outcomes.

Consult, Consent, and Preparation

Symptoms associated with leiomyomata can also be caused by other processes. It is essential that patients undergo preprocedural evaluation to confirm that symptoms are caused by leiomyomata or significantly contributed to by the presence of leiomyomata. It is also critical that more ominous processes (such as ovarian malignancy) be excluded.

The patient should have a normal Papanicolaou (PAP) test result within 12 months before UAE. Patients with abnormal Papanicolaou test results should be referred to their gynecologic care provider for follow-up evaluation and treatment prior to the interventional procedure.

Patients who have continuous bleeding, very prolonged menstrual periods, significant intermenstrual bleeding, or bleeding after menopause may be at increased risk for endometrial hyperplasia or endometrial malignancy. Postmenopausal bleeding is rarely due to fibroids and always warrants endometrial biopsy to rule out malignancy. Similarly, patients with marked irregularity in menstrual bleeding, more frequent than every 21 days or lasting longer than 10 days, should be considered for endometrial biopsy. Communication with the patient's gynecologic care provider is important, as it optimizes outcomes and improves patient care.

Ideally, the most appropriate management of fibroid disease should be determined by the patient after consultation with a Gynecologist and an Interventional Radiologist.

A clinic visit is essential for any patient who may be a candidate for UAE. A complete gynecologic and general medical history should be obtained including symptoms, pregnancy history, history of pelvic infection, results of a recent Papanicolaou (PAP) test or other pathologic results, allergies, current medications, and other medical conditions. Patients should have a general physical examination of sufficient detail to exclude other significant illnesses. This examination should include a focused vascular examination.

Given the minimal expense associated with simple laboratory tests and the variability of menstrual histories, a complete blood count (CBC) should be obtained for each patient. At a minimum, a recent complete blood count should be available for patients with heavy menstrual bleeding. For patients with a history suggesting an underlying bleeding disorder that may be contributing to menstrual bleeding or may complicate percutaneous therapy, activated partial thromboplastin time (aPTT/PTT) and prothrombin time (PT) with international normalized ratio (INR) may be measured along with complete blood count. If there is a history suggesting possible renal insufficiency, blood urea nitrogen (BUN) and/or serum creatinine (Cr) levels should be measured.

Evaluation of a patient's reproductive hormone levels is routinely performed at the authors' institution. This includes measuring follicle-stimulating hormone (FSH), luteinizing hormone (LH), and estradiol. This is performed to clinically determine the patient's reproductive, perimenopausal, or menopausal status. Because of the variability in serum follicle-stimulating hormone levels throughout a patient's menstrual cycle and the pulsatile nature of its secretion, measurement of the serum follicle-stimulating hormone level is of uncertain benefit. No general consensus has been reached as to the role of routine hormone assay in patients who will undergo UAE.

A frank discussion of the procedure risks should always be reviewed with the UAE patient.

The risk of ovarian dysfunction is an important subject to cover. The risk of ovarian failure after UAE has been shown to be age related, with the highest rates occurring in patients older than 45 years of age [18]. The FIBROID registry investigators reported that, of the 1701 UAE patients who completed 12 months follow-up, 7.3% had amenorrhea. Two percent were 35–39 years old, 12% were 40–44 years old, 42% were 45–50 years old, and 43% were older than 50 years of age [60].

Direct embolization of the ovarian artery may be necessary as collateral arterial supply to fibroids of the uterus. The risk of impairment to ovarian function by embolization should be specifically discussed with and approved by the patient during preprocedural consultation.

Additional topics to be reviewed with the patient include the utility of UAE in treating women with leiomyomata and coexisting adenomyosis, or with adenomyosis alone.

Although there are reports that suggest moderate clinical response, the utility of UAE has not been established [61, 62].

Leiomyomata play a role in infertility, subfertility, and complications during pregnancy. The patient should be told that the role of UAE in these situations is not well understood. At this time, the SIR task force does not recommend UAE as primary therapy for infertility in patients with leiomyoma who are reasonable candidates for and will accept myomectomy. For patients who desire children in the future, the decision to perform UAE should be made in the context of the patient's extent of disease, response to previous treatments, and the potential for other treatments to control the symptoms without impairing the ability to achieve and maintain a pregnancy to delivery.

Patient Preparation

There are no currently available data to indicate an ideal time for UAE relative to the menstrual cycle. For patients using gonadotropin-releasing hormone agonists and whose therapy with these agents cannot be discontinued as a result of their severity of bleeding, UAE should be performed immediately before a scheduled injection (i.e., at the nadir of circulating drug levels).

Preoperative labs should include baseline complete blood count, basic metabolic panel with creatinine, and protime/prothrombin time.

A pregnancy test may be obtained on the day of the procedure. It is important to rule out pregnancy, as it is an absolute contraindication for the UAE procedure.

Patients should be instructed to take nothing by mouth after midnight prior to the day of their procedure, in order to be ready for sedation. Exceptions are made for oral medications with sips of water that can be taken the morning of the procedure.

While most operators will give patients periprocedure antibiotics, those patients with history of hydrosalpinx may require special consideration. Doxycycline 100 mg p.o. twice daily for 7 days before the procedure has been suggested as a possible regimen for such patients [63].

Technique

Equipment and Materials

The procedure can be done in the Interventional Radiology suite with fluoroscopic capability.

To ensure the best possible success and safety with this procedure, high-quality angiographic equipment should be used. In general, this requires an angiographic unit in a fixed installation, rather than portable C-arm equipment. The equipment must have adjustable collimators. The machine must be capable of serial radiography and digital subtraction. Ideally, the following features should also be present on the angiographic equipment: reduced-dose pulsed or low-dose continuous fluoroscopy and last image hold, both of which are important in reducing radiation exposure; digital arteriographic imaging with a 1,024 matrix size; digital roadmapping; imaging chain suspended from a C-arm, U-arm, or a combination to allow oblique and complex angulation of the fluoroscope; automatic cumulative fluoroscopic timer; mechanism for recording patient radiation dose, such as dose-area product or cumulative dose at the interventional reference point or skin entrance dose.

Ultrasound with a linear array probe is used frequently to gain arterial access.

A power injector is used for rapid contrast infusion during aortogram or pelvic arteriogram.

Contrast Media

Contrast media may be iso-osmolar and nonionic. Several choices are commercially available from a variety of contrast manufacturers.

Catheters and Wires

Standard access, sheath, catheter, and wire materials include a 4 or 5 French (Fr) Micropuncture® Access Set (Cook Medical Inc, Bloomington, IN), 5 Fr vascular sheath, .035 hydrophilic wire, .035 Bentson wire, a 4 or 5 Fr flush catheter, and any 4 or 5 Fr hockey stick directional catheter. There is a vast array of selective catheters available, and ultimately the operator should simply use whichever one with which he or she is most comfortable. Examples include the 4 or 5 Fr Cobra catheter (Cook Medical Inc, Bloomington, IN) or the 4 or 5 Fr JB1 glide catheter (Cook Medical Inc, Bloomington, IN).

Many operators prefer the 5 Fr Roberts Uterine Artery Catheter (RUC) (Cook Medical Inc, Bloomington, IN), which was specifically designed for this procedure. The catheter has a preformed reverse angle curve at its midshaft and can also function like a Waltman loop. This catheter's unique shape allows it to be seated over the aortic bifurcation, allowing for selection of the contralateral internal iliac artery, and then the uterine artery.

The use of a microcatheter is preferred by some operators. The microcatheter should have a sufficient inner diameter in order to deploy the embolic agent of choice. Examples of possible microcatheters include the 2.4–3 Fr Renegade® Hi Flo™ Microcatheter (Boston Scientific, Natick, MA) with a 0.027 in. inner diameter and the 2.4–2.8 Fr Progreat™ microcatheter (Terumo, Somerset, NJ) with a 0.027 diameter.

The microcatheter is advanced over a 0.018 or 0.014 microwire. Examples of microwires, which may be used include the hydrophilic Terumo glide wire® GT 0.018 wire (Terumo, Somerset, NJ), the Segway® GT 0.014 wire (Biosphere Medical Inc, Rockland, MA), the hydrophilic Transend® EX/Syncho® 0.014 wire (Boston Scientific Corp, Natick, MA), and the Fathom® 0.016 or 0.014 wire (Boston Scientific Corp, Natick, MA).

Embolic Agents

The desired level of arterial occlusion in UAE is quite distal: at the perforating branches. Proximal occlusion of larger arteries with coils or similar agents would not definitively provide clinical success. At present, distal embolization can best be accomplished with particulate agents. Those in current use include polyvinyl alcohol (PVA), tris-acryl gelatin microspheres, and gelatin sponge particles. The latter agent is not approved by the US Food and Drug Administration (FDA) for intra-arterial use, but is commonly employed in this off-label capacity. Polyvinyl alcohol and gelatin microspheres are approved by the FDA for intra-arterial use, but the indication for polyvinyl alcohol is for neurovascular lesions. Gelatin microspheres have a specific indication for use in UAE. Despite these differences in approval status, all three agents appear to be equally safe and effective. It should also be noted that gelatin sponge is considered a temporary embolic agent, whereas PVA and tris-acryl gelatin microspheres are considered permanent embolic agents.

Vascular Closure Devices

Several different vascular closure devices (VCD) are available. The use and choice of VCD should be left to the operator. At the authors' institution, VCDs are used routinely post UAE. Some critics argue that since arterial access is rather small (typically 5 Fr), the patients are not anticoagulated, and frequently the patients are admitted for observation, manual pressure would be the safest route to achieve hemostasis.

Procedure Start

Most centers use conscious sedation to assure patient comfort during the embolization procedure. Each angiographic section that uses conscious sedation must adhere to the conscious sedation policy of its own institution. This is usually a combination of midazolam and fentanyl, with the possible addition of diphenhydramine. There are some operators that prefer epidural or spinal analgesia. General anesthesia is neither required nor recommended.

At the authors' institution, prior to embolizing each uterine artery, ketorolac (Toradol®, Roche, Indiananpolis, IN) 30 mg is given intraveneously (possible 60 mg total dose) to assist in pain management.

Although infectious complications have been reported in the periprocedural interval, the question of antibiotic prophylaxis for uterine artery embolization continues to be debated in the literature. There is little evidence from randomized controlled clinical trials. The clinical practice guidelines set forth by the Society of Interventional Radiology Standards of Practice Committee does recommend routine antibiotic prophylaxis for uterine artery embolization [63]. Although prophylactic antibiotics are commonly given, there is also no consensus as to which agents should be used. At the authors' institution, cefazolin 1 g intravenous is given for the embolization procedure as well as the use of a vascular closure device.

Since the patient and operator are exposed to ionizing radiation during UAE, all procedures must be governed by the principle of "As Low As Reasonably Achievable (ALARA)." The fluoroscopy time and dose should be recorded. The authors routinely dictate this information in the procedure report. This is particularly of concern for women who require the UAE procedure but wish to retain their fertility.

Nausea is a common side effect of the procedure and/or the medications used for pain control. Some practices have advocated prophylactic use of antiemetic agents, whereas others use an "as-needed" approach. Ondansetron may be given intravenously prior to, during, and following the procedure.

The patient is positioned supine, and both groins are prepped with an alcohol or iodophor solution. A sterile drape is placed over the patient for the procedure.

Step by Step

Most operators use a single femoral access site for UAE, whereas others have advocated bilateral access. Some Interventional Radiologists may alternatively use an axillary, brachial, or radial approach. There are no data to indicate that any one of these routes is safer or more efficacious than the other. The choice of an access site (or sites) should be made based on the vascular anatomy of the patient as well as the operator's personal preference.

Figure 1.4a–d demonstrates uterine artery embolization. A flush catheter can be advanced to the abdominal aorta and contrast injection performed with a power injector for abdominal aortogram and pelvic arteriogram (Fig. 1.4a). The abdominal aortogram is helpful in searching for collateral arterial pathways, especially in patients who have a markedly enlarged fibroid uterus. The pelvic arteriogram will map out the course of the internal iliac arteries and the uterine arteries for catheter selection. Some operators suggest obtaining the abdominal aortogram at the end of embolization or, alternatively, at a later date only if the degree of clinical improvement is less than anticipated.

Selection of the contralateral uterine artery (usually left uterine artery from the right groin access) is easier than the side ipsilateral to the groin access (Fig. 1.5). The 4 or 5 Fr directional catheter is advanced to the uterine artery over a 0.035 guide wire of choice. Imaging with the fluoroscope in the contralateral oblique projection will help with visualization of the precise arterial origin. When the catheter tip is seated in the transverse portion of the uterine artery, one may begin to deploy the embolic agent.

Successful treatment of uterine leiomyomata requires distal occlusion of all branches feeding the uterine leiomyomata. Therefore, both uterine arteries should be catheterized and treated unless there are congenital or postoperative variants that prevent bilateral treatment (Fig. 1.4b).

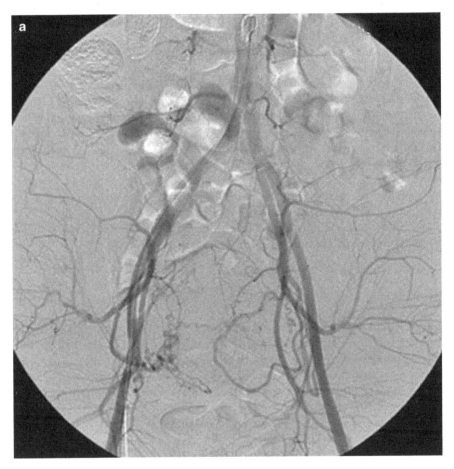

Fig. 1.4 (a–d) Uterine artery embolization. (a) The uterine arteries are enlarged and tortuous. This is typical of the fibroid uterus. (b) Catheter selection to the ipsilateral (right) uterine artery. The catheter tip is in the transverse segment of the artery. The left side has already been embolized. (c) Stasis in the right uterine artery with embolization. (d) Final abdominal aortogram shows no flow in the uterine arteries. There are no collateral arteries to the uterus

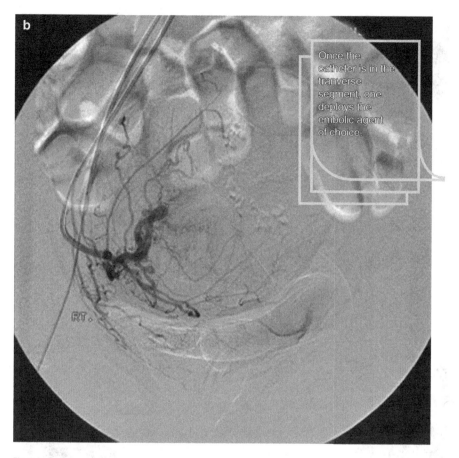

Fig. 1.4 (continued)

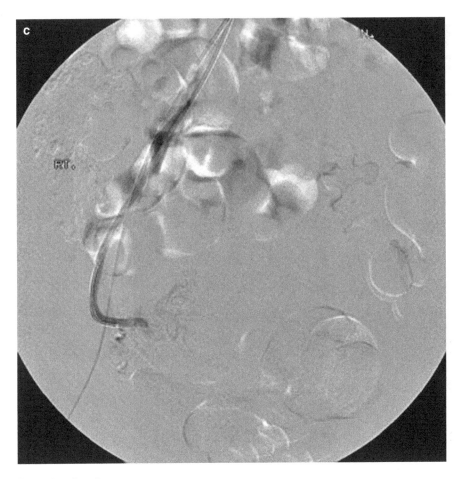

Fig. 1.4 (continued)

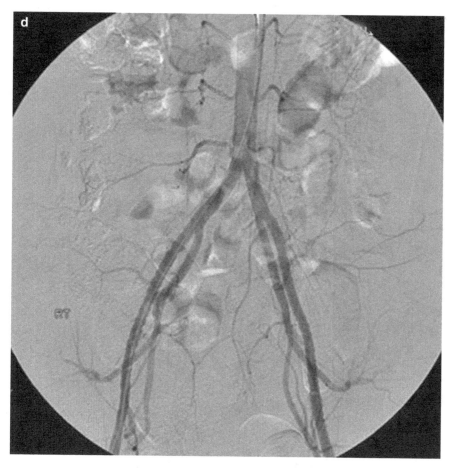

Fig. 1.4 (continued)

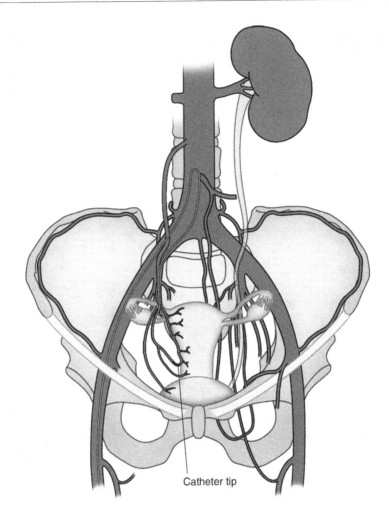

Catheter tip

Fig. 1.5 Catheter selection of the right uterine artery

There is general consensus that UAE performed with polyvinyl alcohol or gelatin sponge particles should be continued until there is complete occlusion of flow in the main uterine artery. Similarly, there is general consensus that UAE performed with gelatin microspheres can be terminated when the branch arteries penetrating the leiomyoma have been occluded, even if significant antegrade flow is still present in the main uterine artery and its first branches. However, it should be noted that these suggested endpoints are based on clinical observation rather than randomized trials (Fig. 1.4c).

Once the desired endpoint of embolization is met, a final abdominal aortogram is performed to verify completion of embolotherapy (Fig. 1.4d). This image should be reviewed for evidence of any collateral arterial flow to the uterus, and a determination made whether to treat collateral arteries.

All catheters, wires, and access sheath may be removed, and attention directed at groin hemostasis. Manual compression is the gold standard, but does require that the patient lay flat for a longer period of time. A vascular closure device (VSD) may be used, and may be particularly helpful in a patient that is obese, hypertensive, or noncompliant. Careful evaluation of the puncture site with a limited femoral arteriogram through the access sheath prior to its removal will provide for proper safe placement of the VSD.

Technical Points, Pitfalls, and Pearls

Patients and treating physicians must be mindful of the radiation dose during UAE, especially for those patients who wish to retain their reproductive potential. Radiation exposure to the patient is directly impacted by technical factors under the operator's control. Although each individual case is unique and may require specific imaging configurations for success, there are several variables that increase patient dose, and they should be used only as necessary to assure technical success: multiple and prolonged image acquisition; image magnification; oblique angulation of the imaging chain; large fields of view (inadequate collimation); large air gap between the patient and the image intensifier; specific types of roadmap imaging (specifically, which may, without notification, disable pulsed or low-dose fluoroscopy).

Some operators inject 5 ml of 1% lidocaine into the uterine artery before embolization. This is done because intra-arterial lidocaine is believed to be a reliable vasodilator and provides an anesthetic effect during embolization procedures and routine angiography [64, 65]. However, it should be noted that Spies et al. found that intra-arterial lidocaine caused significant and diffuse spasm of the uterine artery during their series [66].

There is no current consensus regarding the appropriateness and timing for treating collateral blood supply. Whether sought directly after uterine artery embolization or at a later date, a full abdominal aortogram is necessary to visualize ovarian and lumbar collateral arterial supply to the uterus (Fig. 1.6). Large uterine leiomyomata may receive

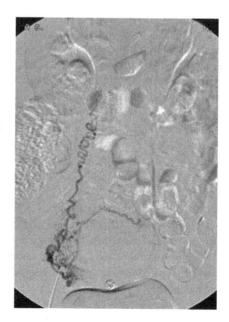

Fig. 1.6 Selective angiogram of the right ovarian artery. Ovarian artery collateral arterial flow is present to the fibroid uterus

collateral blood supply from any pelvic arteries or through adhesions from adjacent pelvic structures. The likelihood of clinical success after UAE will be reduced if the collateral vessels are not recognized and treated. In many but not all cases, embolic occlusion of the collateral supply can be accomplished without significant risk to adjacent structures.

The Interventional Radiologist should be aware that there is a dose–response effect between the amount of embolic used and the risks for complications and pain [67]. (See Complications section of this chapter.) Larger doses may be necessary to achieve symptomatic pain relief in patients who have very large myomata, but this reality should be tempered by the possibility of postoperative problems. Consequently, that patient should be monitored more closely postoperatively in anticipation of any problematic issues.

Postoperative Care, Discharge Instructions, and Follow-Up

Ideally, the patient should be admitted and clinically managed by the Interventional Radiologist performing the procedure. If admitting privileges are not available to the Interventionalist, the patient should be admitted by a Gynecologist or Hospitalist familiar with post UAE patient care.

During hospitalization, most patient-care issues will revolve around pain and nausea management. Clinical inpatient management is very similar to that of other embolotherapy procedures. In some centers, the initiation of pain management may require consultation with an Anesthesiologist and/or a pain service. The Interventional Radiologist should be familiar with post-procedure pain control techniques and use of patient-controlled analgesia (PCA) pumps.

Pain Management

Following UAE, the patient may develop moderate to severe pelvic pain and/or cramping that may last hours. It is essential that there be an appropriate pain management strategy. At the authors' institution, the patient's pain is evaluated before and after the procedure using an analog pain scale. The patient has the use of a PCA pump, usually with morphine at a dose of 0.02 mg/kg, with a 6 min lockout. If fentanyl is to be used, a dose of 0.2 mcg/kg, with a 6 min lockout, is administered.

At this time, there is no consensus regarding the best method of pain management. Patient-controlled analgesia with use of intravenous morphine, meperidine, hydrocodone, or fentanyl has been used effectively in most centers. Others use epidural analgesia, with either a single dose of long-acting narcotic or a continuous infusion of analgesia. Still others prefer use of spinal analgesia. Finally, some operators have used and advocate all oral medication regimens.

Anti-inflammatory medication may assist in the pain control of the post UAE patient. Some possible NSAID choices include ketorolac or diclofenac. The additional use of a steroid such as dexamethasone has been described [68].

Whatever methods and medications are used, each group offering the UAE procedure must be prepared with an approach that can be instituted immediately after the procedure and monitored for adequacy.

Assessing the Need for Hospital Admission

In many interventional practices, UAE is followed by overnight observation in a hospital setting. The purpose of this admission is to assure adequate access to pain and antinausea medications. However, many practices have been successful in discharging patients the day of the procedure. The decision regarding discharge must be made on a case-by-case basis, and should be based on the patient's level of comfort rather than the potential difficulty of arranging an admission. For interventional radiology practices that are not physically connected to a hospital, a mechanism for transferring to a hospital those patients needing admission should be in place before patients are treated. As mentioned previously, Interventional Radiologists who do not have admitting privileges should have in place a mechanism for having patients admitted by another physician who is familiar with the patient. All patients should successfully complete a trial of pain control with oral agents before leaving the hospital.

Inpatient Care

A member of the Interventional Radiology team must be available by telephone or pager during the patient's hospitalization. This is true regardless of the service to which the patient has been admitted. The patient should be evaluated by the operating physician within several hours of completing the procedure to assess adequacy of pain control and to evaluate for any procedure-related complications. The patient must also be evaluated by the operating physician before discharge and be given instructions for home care and follow-up. Written discharge instructions should be provided for the patient. Although nurse practitioners or physician assistants may assist with hospital care, the operating physician should take a leading role in this process and, in particular, discuss with the patient (and family members when appropriate) the outcome of the procedure and anticipated post-procedural course.

Care After Discharge

Oral anti-inflammatory agents and narcotics are commonly used for several days after the procedure. Each group performing UAE should have a post-procedural management strategy developed to provide for pain and nausea control after discharge.

As part of the management plan, each patient should be contacted 24–48 h after discharge to determine the adequacy of pain and nausea control and to screen for any potential early complications.

The patient must have a telephone number for 24 h contact with a member of the team caring for the patient. An Interventional Radiologist must be available for patient consultation during the patient's recovery period. The interventional team should be the point of first contact for problems that the patient may encounter.

If possible, the patient should return for a follow-up outpatient visit 1–3 weeks after the procedure. At this visit, healing of the puncture site(s) may be confirmed, screening for unusual symptoms or potential problems is completed, and the patient may be reinstructed on subsequent follow-up plans.

Physicians performing UAE must be prepared to provide long-term follow-up for their patients. This is important for monitoring the control of symptoms, but also for detecting complications that may occur. Late infections, expulsion of portions of leiomyomata, chronic endometritis, chronic vaginal discharge, and cessation or irregularity of menses have all been described after UAE and may develop more than a year after the procedure.

Follow-up imaging is indicated 6–12 months after the procedure (Fig. 1.7a–d). This is useful in determining whether existing leiomyomata have been infarcted and are decreasing in volume. Follow-up imaging will also help determine whether any uterine or adnexal complications have occurred. In addition, post-procedure imaging provides a "new baseline" measurement of leiomyoma volume against which any subsequent increase in size (which might indicate leiomyosarcoma) can be compared.

Repeat Treatment

Inadequate clinical improvement or volume reduction on follow-up imaging may lead to a second angiographic examination and repeat embolization. This may be appropriate if, on imaging studies, there is evidence of continued perfusion of the leiomyomata. Alternatively, if all the visualized lesions demonstrate fibrotic change and an absence of perfusion, repeat treatment is unlikely to be of use. MR imaging with contrast is of particular utility in making this determination.

If repeat treatment is performed, it should be preceded by a discussion with the patient that specifically addresses the risks of ovarian injury. This discussion is important because ovarian collateral supply is a common cause for treatment failure, and more aggressive embolization during a second treatment may theoretically result in ovarian injury and cause accelerated ovarian failure.

Outcomes

The technical success rate for successful embolization of both uterine arteries is 96% [69]. However, the measure of UAE efficacy is the degree to which symptoms and quality of life is improved after the procedure. Prion et al. reported a 91% rate of patient satisfaction with UAE in short-term follow-up. Eighty-three percent of patients reported improvement in menorrhagia, 77% in dysmenorrhea, 84% in bulk-related symptoms, and 86% in urinary symptoms 3 months after UAE [70].

Pelage et al. showed significant improvement in UAE patients at intermediate-term follow-up (17 months). The vast majority of women in their patient cohort reported significant improvement in all fibroid-related symptoms. Menorrhagia improved in 84%, bulk-related symptoms in 82%, and menstrual pain in 79%. Only 3% of patients had severe symptoms that failed to respond. The vast majority of patients stated that they would undergo repeat embolization if deemed medically necessary [19].

The longest post UAE follow-up published is by Spies et al. One hundred and eighty-two patients were followed 5 years post UAE. Seventy-three percent of patients reported symptom improvement at 5 years, with 76% reporting continued satisfaction with the procedure in this interval [71].

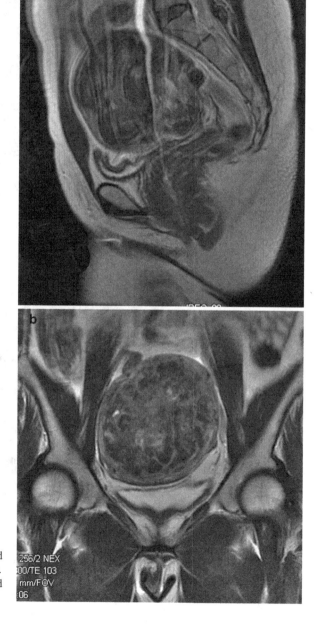

Fig. 1.7 (a–d) MRI pelvis pre- and post-uterine artery embolization. The patient's follow-up study was obtained 6 months after the procedure. Note the change in signal and decreased volume

Fig. 1.7 (continued)

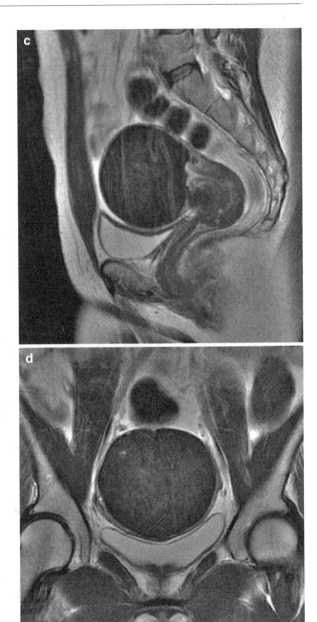

The FIBROID registry presented clinical outcomes of UAE in a wide variety of centers. Seventy-two patients enrolled in the registry within the US and internationally. Three thousand and five patients were originally registered, with 30 day follow-up performed in 2,729. Of the women that were enrolled, 1,701 completed 1 year follow-up. Eighty-seven percent of patients had a significant improvement in symptoms score; less than 6% had no improvement in symptoms. Eighty-two percent of patients reported satisfaction with the procedure at 12 months [72].

The distinction between adenomyosis and leiomyomata is of clinical importance, as clinical outcomes with uterine artery embolization vary. A few studies have reported durable improvement in symptoms in 50–70% of patients with adenomyosis alone or coexistent adenomyosis and leiomyomata [61]. Although hysterectomy is frequently required for recurrent symptoms in up to 50% of patients within 3 years of embolization, UAE can still be considered a reasonable option in patients that desire fertility, are high risk for surgery, or desire uterine preservation [62].

Potentially, UAE may have an adverse effect on future fertility. At the authors' institution, FSH levels are obtained, typically on the third day of the menstrual cycle. Elevated FSH levels indicate loss of functional ovarian reserve. Several studies have shown no permanent decline in ovarian function, up to 12 months [73–75]. Though there have been anecdotal reports of increased rates of breech delivery, two large studies have recently shown nonconsistent antenatal or peripartum complications post UAE [76, 77]. Despite the findings of these studies, at our institution, the patient is routinely counseled that fertility outcomes cannot be predicted with certainty and may depend on the type and extent of fibroid disease. Since more is known about pregnancy outcomes post myomectomy, the authors usually recommend myomectomy if the patient wishes to become pregnant within 2 years. That being said, in select cases, UAE can still be considered in those patients wishing to become pregnant but have diffuse disease (poor candidate for myomectomy), have failed prior myomectomy, and have no immediate plans to become pregnant.

Complications

Uterine fibroid embolization is a generally uncomplicated procedure with a short hospital stay and low incidence of adverse events. An adverse event is one in which a patient is required to stay in the hospital for more than 48 h after initial hospitalization, if the patient must visit the emergency room, or if the patient must return to the hospital for readmission following the procedure [78]. One study found a major adverse event rate of 0.66% in the hospital and 4.8% within 30 days of the procedure [78]. Another study, based on a review of the literature, reported four deaths related to UAE: two from pulmonary embolus and two from septicemia [79, 80].

The most common complications are pain, bleeding, or infection associated with the passage of an embolized fibroid. Volkers et al. showed a strong dose–response effect between the amount of embolization material used and the occurrence of pain, fever, and short-term complications [67]. No life-threatening complications were seen in that study.

The complication of necrotic fibroid passage tended to occur with intracavitary or partially intracavitary fibroids that have a shared interface with the endometrial cavity. This can occur in up to 5% of the patient population following UAE [81, 82]. During the process of fibroid passage, portions of necrotic fibroid tissue may remain attached to the endometrium causing a nidus for infection. Cramping and bleeding may also occur as the tissue is passed with the level of discomfort proportional to the size of the fibroid.

Necrotic tissue may pass spontaneously. If not, gynecologic intervention may be required (e.g., performance of a dilatation and curettage).

Unintentional, or non-target, embolization of the ovarian artery may result from collateral blood circulation of ovarian vessels from the uterine artery, which has been reported in up to 11% of the population [83]. It should be emphasized that this risk is theoretical and does not occur in all patients who have uterine artery embolization performed. If there is specific concern as to the patency of the ovarian vessels, Doppler US or angiography may be used to assess flow through the ovarian vessels following embolization of the uterine arteries.

As mentioned earlier, ovarian dysfunction leading to transient or permanent amenorrhea may occur as well. This may be due to, or at least partially attributed to, the effect of non-target embolization [78]. In a 2004 study of 102 patients undergoing UAE, six had new onset amenorrhea up to 3 months after procedure, with an age range of 38–48 years. An additional six patients had new onset amenorrhea by 12 months, all of whom were 45 years or older [78].

As with all interventional procedures, puncture site injuries causing neurovascular complications may occur, although these are rare. Venous thromboembolic events (VTE) may occur in UAE patients as with other surgical patients. In general, patients who smoke or use oral contraceptives are at higher risk for VTE.

Summary and Conclusions

Since it was first reported in the literature, UAE has rapidly evolved to a standard-of-care treatment option in the clinical management of women with symptomatic uterine leiomyomata. The procedure has been evaluated in many clinical series around the world and found to be safe and effective. Clinical response rates have been shown to vary between 80 and 90%, with an overall complication rate of less than 3% [19, 70, 71]. The success of the procedure has generated incredible interest among patients and has been widely reported in the lay press and on the Internet.

UAE, aside from offering the patient a documented and beneficial treatment, has ushered in a new era in Interventional Radiology. The procedure, though well within the professional scope of Interventional Radiologists, requires patient care skills that must be clinically developed and fostered. Complete patient care, from the initial patient encounter in clinic through the actual procedure to the long-term follow-up, demands the full involvement of the Interventional Radiologist in order to achieve true clinical success.

References

1. Mäkinen J, Johansson J, Tomás C, et al. Morbidity of 10,110 hysterectomies by type of approach. Hum Reprod. 2001;16:1473–8.
2. Reed S, Newton K, Thompson L, et al. The incidence of repeat uterine surgery following myomectomy. J Womens Health. 2006;15(9):1046–52.

3. Goodwin SC, Vedantham S, McLucas B, et al. Preliminary experience with uterine artery embolization for uterine fibroids. J Vasc Interv Radiol. 1997;8:517–26.
4. ACOG Issues Opinion on Uterine Artery Embolization for Treatment of Fibroids. Presented at the American College of Obstetricians and Gynecologists annual clinical meeting, Philadelphia, PA. May 1–5, 2004.
5. Pelage J, Julien C, Etienne P, et al. Uterine fibroid vascularization and clinical relevance to uterine fibroid embolization. Radiographics. 2005;25(special issue):99–117.
6. Ligon A, Morton C. Leiomyomata: treatability and cytogenetic studies. Human Reproduction Update 2008;7:8.
7. Ligon A, Morton C. Genetics of uterine leiomyomata. Genes Chromosomes Cancer. 2000;28:235.
8. Baird D, Dunson DB, Hill MC, et al. High cumulative incidence of uterine leiomyoma in black and white women: ultrasound evidence. Am J Obstet Gynecol. 2003;188:100–7.
9. Rackow B, Arici A. Fibroids and in-vitro fertilization: which comes first? Curr Opin Obstet Gynecol. 2005;17:225–31.
10. Lumsden M, Wallace E. Clinical presentation of uterine fibroids. Baillieres Clin Obstet Gynaecol. 1998;12:177–95.
11. Uflacker R. Atlas of vascular anatomy. 2nd ed. Philadelphia: Lippincott Williams & Wilkins; 2007. p. 655–79.
12. Gomez-Jorge J, Keyoung A, Levy E, et al. Uterine artery anatomy relevant to uterine leiomyomata embolization. Cardiovasc Intervent Radiol. 2003;26:522–7.
13. Yeagley T, Goldberg J, Klein T, et al. Labial necrosis after uterine artery embolization for leiomyomata. Obstet Gynecol. 2002;100(5 part 1):881–2.
14. Vott S, Bonilla S, Goodwin S, et al. CT findings after uterine artery embolization. J Comput Assist Tomogr. 2000;24:846–8.
15. Ghai S, Rajan D, Benjamin M, Asch M, Gahi S. Uterine artery embolization for leiomyomas: pre and post procedural evaluation with US. Radiographics. 2005;25:1159–76.
16. Lev-Toaff A, Toaff M, Liu J, et al. Value of sonohysterography in the diagnosis and management of abnormal uterine bleeding. Radiology. 1996;201:179–84.
17. Becker Jr E, Lev-Toaff A, Kaufmann E, et al. The added value of transvaginal sonohysterography over transvaginal sonography alone in women with known or suspected leiomyoma. J Ultrasound Med. 2002;21:237–47.
18. Fedele L, Bianchi S, Dorta M, Brioschi D, et al. Transvaginal ultrasonography versus hysteroscopy in the diagnosis of uterine submucosal myomas. Obstet Gynecol. 1991;77:745–8.
19. Pron G, Bennett J, Common A, et al. The Ontario Uterine Fibroid Embolization Trial II. Uterine fibroid reduction and symptom relief after uterine artery embolization for fibroids. Fertil Steril. 2003;79:120–7.
20. Tranquart F, Brunereau L, Cottier J, et al. Prospective sonographic assessment of uterine artery embolization for the treatment of fibroids. Ultrasound Obstet Gynecol. 2002;19:81–7.
21. Goodwin S, Bonilla S, Sacks D, et al. Reporting standards for uterine artery embolization for the treatment of uterine leiomyomata. J Vasc Intervent Radiol. 2001;12:1011–20.
22. Ascher S, Arnold L, Patt R, et al. Adenomyosis: prospective comparison of MR imaging and transvaginal sonography. Radiology. 1994;190:803–6.
23. Togashi K, Ozasa H, Konishi I, et al. Enlarged uterus: differentiation between adenomyosis and leiomyoma with MR imaging. Radiology. 1989;171:531–4.
24. Reinhold C, Tafazoli F, Mehio A, et al. Uterine adenomyosis: endovaginal US and MR imaging features with histopathologic correlation. Radiographics. 1999;19:147–60.
25. Atri M, Reinhold C, Mehio A, Chapman W, et al. Adenomyosis: US features with histologic correlation in an in vitro study. Radiology. 2000;215:783–90.
26. Imaoka I, Wada A, Matsuo M, Yoshida M, et al. MR imaging of disorders associated with female infertility: use in diagnosis, treatment, and management. Radiographics. 2003;23:1401–21.

27. McLucas B, Perrella R, Goodwin S, et al. Role of uterine artery Doppler flow in fibroid embolization. J Ultrasound Med. 2002;21:113–20.
28. Weintraub J, Romano W, Kirsch M, Sam-paleanu D, et al. Uterine artery embolization: sonographic imaging findings. J Ultrasound Med. 2002;21:633–7.
29. Nicholson T, Pelage J, Ettles D. Fibroid calcification after uterine artery embolization: ultrasonographic appearance and pathology. J Vasc Interv Radiol. 2001;12:443–6.
30. Mayer D, Shipilov V. Ultrasonography and magnetic resonance imaging of uterine fibroids. Obstet Gynecol Clin North Am. 1995;22:667–725.
31. Hricak H, Tscholakoff D, Heinrichs L, et al. Uterine leiomyomas: correlation of MR, histopathologic findings, and symptoms. Radiology. 1986;158:385–91.
32. Dudiak C, Turner D, Patel C, et al. Uterine leiomyomas in the infertile patient: preoperative localization with MR imaging versus US and hysterosalpingography. Radiology. 1988;167:627–30.
33. Zawin M, McCarthy S, Scoutt L, et al. High-field MRI and US evaluation of the pelvis in women with leiomyomas. Magn Reson Imaging. 1990;8:371–6.
34. Prayson R, Hart W. Pathologic considerations of uterine smooth muscle tumors. Obstet Gynecol Clin North Am. 1995;22:637–57.
35. Yamashita Y, Torashima M, Takahashi M, et al. Hyperintense uterine leiomyoma at T2-weighted MR imaging: differentiation with dynamic enhanced MR imaging and clinical implications. Radiology. 1993;189:721–5.
36. Okizuka H, Sugimura K, Takemori M, et al. MR detection of degenerating uterine leiomyomas. J Comput Assist Tomogr. 1993;17:760–6.
37. Kawakami S, Togashi K, Konishi I, et al. Red degeneration of uterine leiomyoma: MR appearance. J Comput Assist Tomogr. 1994;18:925–8.
38. Bradley Jr WG. MR appearance of hemorrhage in the brain. Radiology. 1993;189:15–26.
39. Mittl Jr RL, Yeh IT, Kressel HY. High signal intensity rim surrounding uterine leiomyomas on MR images; pathologic correlation. Radiology. 1991;180:81–3.
40. Novak E. Novak's gynecologic and obstetric pathology. 8th ed. Philadelphia: Saunders; 1979. p. 280–90.
41. Mark AS, Hricak H, Heinrichs LW, et al. Adenomyosis and leiomyoma: differential diagnosis with MR imaging. Radiology. 1987;163:527–9.
42. Togashi K, Nishimura K, Itoh K, et al. Adenomyosis: diagnosis with MR imaging. Radiology. 1988;166:111–4.
43. Reinhold C, McCarthy S, Bret P, et al. Diffuse adenomyosis: comparison of endovaginal US and MR imaging with histopathologic correlation. Radiology. 1996;199:151–8.
44. Outwater E, Siegelman E, Van Deerlin V. Adenomyosis; current concepts and imaging considerations. AJR Am J Roentgenol. 1998;170:437–41.
45. Weinreb J, Barkoff N, Megibow A, et al. The value of MR imaging in distinguishing leiomyomas from other solid pelvic masses when sonography is indeterminate. AJR Am J Roentgenol. 1990;154:295–9.
46. Troiano R, Lazzarini K, Scoutt L, et al. Fibroma and fibrothecoma of the ovary: MR imaging findings. Radiology. 1997;204:795–8.
47. Outwater EK, Eigelman ES, Kim B, et al. Ovarian Brenner tumors: MR imaging characteristics. Magn Reson Imaging. 1998;16:1147–53.
48. Keir R, McCarthy SM, Scoutt LM, et al. Pelvic masses in pregnancy: MR imaging. Radiology. 1990;176:709–13.
49. Togashi K, Kawakami S, Kimura I, et al. Uterine contractions: possible diagnostic pitfall at MR imaging. J Magn Reson Imaging. 1993;2:889–93.
50. Togashi K, Kawakami S, Kimura I, et al. Sustained uterine contractions: a cause of hypointense myometrial bulging. Radiology. 1993;187:707–10.
51. Pattani SJ, Kier R, Deal R, Luchansky E. MRI of uterine leiomyosarcoma. Magn Reson Imaging. 1995;12:331–3.

52. Leibsohn S, d'Ablaing G, Mishell Jr DR, Schlaerth JB. Leiomyosarcoma in a series of hysterectomies performed for presumed uterine leiomyomas. Am J Obstet Gynecol. 1990; 162:968–76.
53. Parker W, Fu Y, Berek J. Uterine sarcoma in patients operated on for presumed leiomyoma and rapidly growing leiomyoma. Obstet Gynecol. 1994;83:414–8.
54. Andrews R, Spies J, Sacks D, et al. Patient care and uterine artery embolization for leiomyomata. J Vasc Interv Radiol. 2009;20(7):S307–11.
55. McLucas B, Goodwin S, Adler L, et al. Pregnancy following uterine fibroid embolization. Int J Gynaecol Obstet. 2001;74:1–7.
56. Ravina J, Vigneron N, Aymard A, et al. Pregnancy after embolization of uterine myoma: report of 12 cases. Fertil Steril. 2000;73:1241–3.
57. Mara M, Maskova J, Fucikova Z, et al. Midterm clinical and first reproductive results of a randomized controlled trial comparing uterine fibroid embolization and myomectomy. Cardiovasc Intervent Radiol. 2008;31:73–85.
58. Usadi R, Marshburn PB. The impact of uterine artery embolization on fertility and pregnancy outcome. Curr Opin Obstet Gynecol. 2007;19:279–83.
59. Holub Z, Mara M, Kuzel D, et al. Pregnancy outcomes after uterine artery occlusion: prospective multicentric study. Fertil Steril. 2008;90:1886–91.
60. Verma S, Bergin D, Gonsalves C, et al. Submucosal fibroids becoming endocavitary following uterine artery embolization: risk assessment by MRI. AJR Am J Roentgenol. 2008;190: 1220–6.
61. Spies J, Roth AR, Jha R, et al. Uterine artery embolization for leiomyomata: factors associated with successful symptomatic and imaging outcome. Radiology. 2002;222:45–52.
62. Kim MD, Kim S, Kim NK, et al. Long-term results of uterine artery embolization for symptomatic adenomyosis. AJR Am J Roentgenol. 2007;188:176–81.
63. Goldberg J. Uterine artery embolization for adenomyosis: looking at the glass half full. Radiology. 2005;236:1111–2.
64. Venkatesan A, Kundu S, Sacks D, et al. Practice guideline for adult antibiotic prophylaxis during vascular and interventional radiology procedures. J Vasc Interv Radiol. 2010;21(11): 1611–30.
65. Molgaard CP, Teitelbaum GP, Pentecost MJ, et al. Intraarterial administration of lidocaine for analgesia in hepatic chemoembolization. J Vasc Interv Radiol. 1990;1:81–5.
66. Gordon I, Westcott J. Intra-arterial lidocaine: an effective analgesic for peripheral angiography. Radiology. 1977;124:43–5.
67. Keyoung J, Levy E, Roth A, et al. Intraarterial lidocaine for pain control after uterine artery embolization for leiomyomata. J Vasc Interv Radiol. 2001;12(9):1065–9.
68. Volkers NA, Hehenkamp WJ, Birnie E, et al. Uterine artery embolization in the treatment of symptomatic uterine fibroid tumors (EMMY Trial): periprocedural results and complications. J Vasc Interv Radiol. 2006;17(3):471–80.
69. Lampmann LE, Lohle PN, Smeets A, et al. Management during uterine artery embolization for symptomatic uterine fibroids. Cardiovasc Intervent Radiol. 2007;30(4):809–11.
70. Stokes L, Wallace M, Godwin R, et al. Quality improvement guidelines for uterine artery embolization for symptomatic leiomyomas. J Vasc Interv Radiol. 2010;21(8): 1153–68.
71. Walker WJ, Pelage J. Uterine artery embolization for symptomatic fibroids: clinical results in 400 women with imaging follow up. Br J Obstet Gynaecol. 2002;109:1262–72.
72. Spies J, Bruno J, Czeyda-Pommersheim F, et al. Long-term outcome of uterine artery embolization of leiomyomas. Obstet Gynecol. 2005;106:933–9.
73. Spies JJ, Myers ER, Worthington-Kirsch R, et al. The FIBROID Registry: symptom and quality of life status 1 year after therapy. Obstet Gynecol. 2005;106:1309–18.
74. Healey S, Buzaglo K, Seti L, et al. Ovarian function after uterine artery embolization and hysterectomy. J Am Assoc Gynecol Laparosc. 2004;11:348–52.

75. Speis JB, Roth AR, Gonsalves SM, Murphy-Skryniarz KM. Ovarian function after uterine artery embolization for leiomyomata: assessment with use of serum follicle stimulating hormone assay. J Vasc Interv Radiol. 2001;12:437–42.

76. Tropenano G, Di Stasi C, Litwicka K, et al. Uterine artery embolization for fibroids does not have adverse effects on ovarian reserve in regularly cycling women younger than 40 years. Fertil Steril. 2004;8:1055–61.

77. Carpenter TT, Walker WJ. Pregnancy following uterine artery embolization for symptomatic fibroids: a series of 26 completed pregnancies. Br J Obstet Gynaecol. 2005;112:321–5.

78. Pron G, Mocarski E, Bennett J, et al. Pregnancy after uterine artery embolization for leiomyomata: The Ontario Multicenter Trial. Obstet Gynecol. 2005;105:67–76.

79. Mauro M, Murphy K, Thomson K, et al. Image-guided interventions. 1st ed. Philadelphia: Saunders Elsevier; 2008.

80. Vashisht A, Studd J, Carey A, Burn P. Fatal septicaemia after fibroid embolization. Lancet. 1999;354:307–8.

81. Lanocita R, Frigerio LF, Patelli G et al. A fatal complication of percutaneous transcatheter embolization for the treatment of uterine fibroids. Presented at the SMIT/CIMIT 11th Annual Scientific Meeting, Boston, MA. September 16–18, 1999.

82. Pelage J, Le Dref O, Jacob D, et al. Selective arterial embolization of the uterine arteries in the management of intractable post-partum hemorrhage. Acta Obstet Gynecol Scand. 1999;78:698–703.

83. Andersen PE, Lund N, Justesen P, et al. Uterine artery embolization of symptomatic uterine fibroids. Initial success and short-term results. Acta Radiol. 2001;42:234–8.

84. Pelage J, Le Dref O, Soyer P, et al. Arterial anatomy of the female genital tract: variations and relevance to transcatheter embolization of the uterus. Am J Roentgenol. 1999;172:989–94.

Pelvic Varices Embolization

2

Anthony C. Venbrux, Giriraj K. Sharma, Emily Timmreck Jackson,
Amy P. Harper, and Lena Hover

Introduction

Pelvic venous incompetence (PVI) or pelvic congestion syndrome (PCS) is a disease entity that is characterized by a pain syndrome known as chronic pelvic pain (CPP) and is caused by varices. More broadly, CPP in women is defined as noncyclic pain originating in the lower abdomen or pelvis for more than 6 months in duration [1]. A potentially debilitating condition, CPP is estimated to affect as many as 39.1% of women at some point in their lives [2]. While the etiology of CPP is variable, pelvic venous incompetence (PVI) or pelvic congestion syndrome (PCS) has been recognized as a cause of CPP since 1949 [3]. PVI or PCS is defined as venous incompetence in ovarian, internal iliac, or parauterine veins, resulting in increased venous filling (i.e., congestion or engorgement) and subsequent development of ovarian and internal iliac (i.e., pelvic) varicosities. The term PVI is preferred over the older name, PCS, because it more accurately reflects the pathophysiology associated with the condition.

Pathophysiology

Ovarian varicosities were first described by Richet in 1857 [4]. However, it was not until the late 1920s when Cotte first linked ovarian varicosities in women with CPP, an association supported by Taylor in 1949 [3, 5]. The precise etiology of primary pelvic varices is unknown and likely multifactorial. Mechanical factors such as damaged or absent venous valves are significant in the development of retrograde flow and engorged veins [3].

Considering PVI (PCS) primarily affects young premenopausal women, ovarian activity and hormonal factors may also contribute to the development of varicosities [6]. The ovarian veins are exposed to a 100-fold high concentration of estradiol and estrone compared to the peripheral circulation. Resulting distension of the ovarian veins will worsen symptoms of PVI [7]. Reports of improvement in PVI symptoms when patients reach menopause or undergo hormonal suppression support this concept.

A.C. Venbrux (✉)
Department of Radiology, Division of Interventional Radiology,
The George Washington University Medical Center, Washington, DC, USA
e-mail: avenbrux@mfa.gwu.edu

E.A. Ignacio and A.C. Venbrux (eds.), *Women's Health in Interventional Radiology*,
DOI 10.1007/978-1-4419-5876-1_2, © Springer Science+Business Media, LLC 2012

A summary of causes of pelvic varices described in the literature, in addition to those listed above, include: (a) uterine malposition leading to pelvic vein kinking, (b) hydrostatic causes (e.g., pregnancy), (c) external vascular compression including the renal "Nutcracker" syndrome, (d) portal hypertension, (e) iliac compression syndrome (May-Thurner Syndrome), or (f) inferior vena cava syndrome [6–10].

Clinical Manifestations

PVI typically presents in young, multiparous women in their late 20s or early 30s [8, 11]. Commonly reported symptoms include a deep, dull pelvic ache, dyspareunia, and postcoital pain. Dull pain is usually present in the lower pelvis, the vulvar region, and the thighs. Sharp exacerbations occur after walking, prolonged standing, or activities that increase intra-abdominal pressure (lifting or bearing down). Patients often feel best in the morning. Pain is typically worse at the end of the day, during the premenstrual period, and/or during pregnancy [6, 7]. The condition may worsen after each subsequent pregnancy. On physical examination, the patient may have visible varicosities in the pudendal, vulvar, and labial regions.

Anatomy

Veins of the Pelvis

Anatomy of the pelvic venous outflow is variable. On the left, venous drainage from the pelvis is predominantly via the *left ovarian vein* and the *left internal iliac vein*. The left ovarian vein empties into the left renal vein (Fig. 2.1). The left internal iliac venous plexus drains into the deep pelvic central veins. In females, there is venous communication (blood flow) between the ovarian veins and the internal iliac veins. In addition, there is flow across the midline to the contralateral side as well as communication with veins in the upper thighs, pelvic floor, lower gastrointestinal tract, etc.

On the right side, venous drainage from the *right ovarian vein* empties into the central venous system generally at the junction of the inferior vena cava (IVC) and the right renal vein. The *right internal iliac vein* is similar to the left in its pattern of venous communications.

Anatomic variation in the pelvic venous anatomy is common and may include the finding of multiple dividing split parallel venous trunks comprising the left or right ovarian venous outflow (e.g., a single trunk at the level of the left renal vein with division into multiple trunks in the pelvis). Similarly, there may be duplications in the venous outflow of the internal iliac veins (e.g., two smaller internal trunks on one side of the pelvis rather than a single larger trunk, etc.).

On the left side of the pelvis, the left common iliac vein may be compressed by the crossing right common iliac artery anteriorly and the lumbosacral skeletal structures posteriorly. If significant, this may lead to left-sided pelvic venous outflow obstruction. This clinical entity is known as iliac compression syndrome (May-Thurner Syndrome) and may result in deep venous thrombosis (DVT) (i.e., recurrent left lower extremity DVTs, left leg swelling, and diversion of blood into the left internal iliac vein resulting in pelvic varices).

Fig. 2.1 Anatomy of ovarian
and internal iliac varices

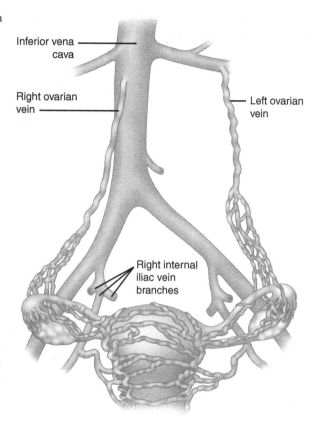

Inferior vena
cava

Right ovarian
vein

Left ovarian
vein

Right internal
iliac vein
branches

Infrequently, the left renal vein may be extrinsically compressed by vascular structures (e.g., retroaortic left renal vein). Compression of venous outflow from the left renal vein then causes elevated venous pressures in the hilum of the left kidney with reversal of blood flow in the left ovarian vein. This retrograde flow may result in large left ovarian veins with associated pelvic pain. This syndrome is called "Nutcracker Syndrome," as the compression of the renal vein between two "pinching" structures (i.e., the aorta anteriorly and the spine posteriorly) is analogous to the compression of a nutcracker.

Valves exist in the main trunks of ovarian veins but generally not in the internal iliac veins. Ovarian vein valvular incompetence may lead to reversal of venous flow in the ovarian vein with venous dilation of veins in the pelvis and development of ovarian and internal iliac varices. Hydrostatic pressure also plays a role, as women with PVI generally note increased pelvic pain with long periods of standing or sitting and report improved pain when supine.

Communications with multiple other venous tributaries in the pelvis may explain, in part, the development of (1) vulvar and vaginal varices (i.e., communication with the internal iliac veins) (Fig. 2.2) and (2) the worsening of varices in the upper thighs, buttocks, and groin areas (i.e., communication of the internal iliac veins with the saphenofemoral junction, etc.). Thus, knowledge of pelvic venous anatomy helps explain clinical conditions such as PVI and helps direct use of endovascular techniques for treatment.

Fig. 2.2 Left internal iliac venogram. There are prominent midline pelvic varicosities with collateralization to perineal/vaginal and vulvar varices

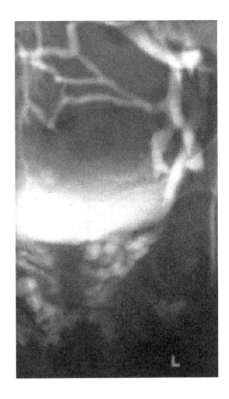

Imaging

When a diagnosis of PVI is clinically considered, noninvasive imaging is the next step to confirm the presence of pelvic varicosities. Pelvic ultrasound (US) is a common first-line choice for investigation and can be conducted transabdominally or transvaginally [12] (Figs. 2.3a–c). Computed tomography (CT) (Fig. 2.4) and magnetic resonance (MR) imaging (Fig. 2.5) depict pelvic varices as tortuous and dilated, enhancing vascular structures in the pelvis. MR imaging is often the diagnostic modality of choice because of its multiplanar imaging capability and lack of ionizing radiation. However, because the patient is supine during CT and MR imaging and generally during US evaluation, pelvic varices may be less prominent. Additionally, ovarian and pelvic varices may not be addressed or diagnosed on supine MR, CT, or US scans because the consideration of this finding as "pathologic" may not be considered in the differential diagnosis of causes for chronic pelvic pain (i.e., a "lack of awareness"). MR and CT scans should be obtained and images depicted in the coronal, axial, and sagittal projections to better define anatomy and to avoid missed diagnoses. Recently, contrast-enhanced magnetic resonance venography (MRV) has gained popularity for diagnosis of PVI.

In the past, laparoscopy was commonly used in the diagnosis of PVI prior to the technologic advancements of noninvasive imaging modalities. Laparoscopic evaluation bears risk of a missed diagnosis of PVI in more than 80% of patients [13]. This is most likely

Fig. 2.3 (a–c) Pelvic
ultrasound shows
robust varices in the
pelvis

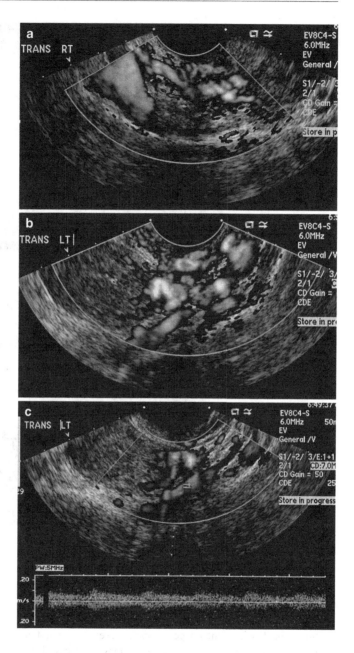

due to patient positioning and instillation of carbon dioxide under pressure during the
laparoscopic evaluation. Venography remains the "gold standard" for diagnosis of PVI.
Venography offers the Interventional Radiologist a detailed depiction of venous anatomy,
including identification of retrograde reflux, contralateral venous filling, internal iliac venous
drainage, and any extension of venous collaterals into the central venous system [6].

Fig. 2.4 CT scan pelvis. There are serpiginous varices posteriorly

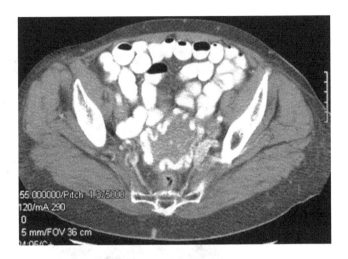

Fig. 2.5 Coronal contrast-enhanced pelvic MRI. Note the serpiginous varices surrounding the pelvic organs

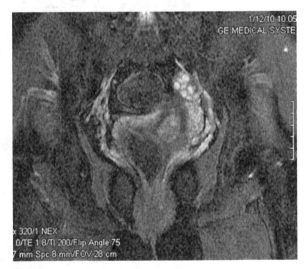

Patient Encounter

Indications and Contraindications

Treatment for PVI in women depends on the severity of symptoms and clinical course of the patient. As reported in the literature, the range of medical therapeutic options is considerable [14]. First-line pharmacologic treatment is the use of analgesics. Other medical treatments of PVI include psychotherapy, progestins, danazol, phlebotonics, gonadotropin releasing hormone (GnRH) agonists with hormone replacement therapy (HRT), dihydro-ergotamine, and nonsteroidal anti-inflammatory drugs. Specifically, the literature supports use of medroxyprogesterone acetate (MPA) or the GnRH analogue goserelin in an effort to suppress ovarian function and/or increase venous contraction. MPA may be given orally

30 mg/day for 6 months. Goserelin acetate is dosed as an injection of 3.6 mg monthly over a 6 month period. As chemical ovarian "ligation" has numerous side effects, estrogen replacement or "add-back" therapy is frequently required as well [15].

If the patient has continued significant symptoms with minimal relief from pharmaco-therapy, hysterectomy with or without bilateral salpingo-oophorectomy has been reported as last resort treatment. Treatment of PVI by hysterectomy, however, is not always cura-tive. Studies show that among patients having undergone hysterectomy for PVI, 33% report residual pain and 20% experience recurrence of disease [16, 17].

In the authors' experience, hysterectomy is often not helpful and is associated with signifi-cant surgical risk. Additionally, many women are appropriately concerned with loss of fertility and the physical and clinical sequelae of a surgical hysterectomy/oophorectomy. Therefore, minimally invasive endovascular techniques remain an important treatment option.

Edwards et al. first introduced transcatheter embolotherapy (TCE) in 1993, a procedure, which has changed the management of women with PVI [18]. With refinement over the past decade, the technique of percutaneous embolization has been shown to improve clini-cal efficacy and reduce morbidity. Following clinical evaluation, screening imaging, stud-ies, and venography, women with a suspected diagnosis of ovarian and internal iliac varices are potential candidates for transcatheter embolotherapy.

Indications for treatment include women with chronic noncyclic pelvic pain for 6 months or more that is not relieved by other medical therapies.

Contraindications for treatment of PVI using transcatheter techniques include active infection (e.g., bacteremia, pelvic inflammatory disease, etc.), allergy to contrast, and severe coagulopathy.

Consult, Consent, and Preparation

The patient should have an appropriate clinical history and imaging prior to the consultation visit. (See previous section in this chapter on Imaging) Appropriate imaging is a priority for pre-procedure planning whenever possible. Imaging is performed not only to document varices but to rule out other potential causes of pelvic pain (e.g., large ovarian cysts, uterine leiomyomata, etc.).

At some institutions, laparoscopy is performed, which again may be "negative" for reasons outlined previously in the Imaging section of this chapter. This is not a requirement at the authors' institution.

Given the complexity of PVI (PCS) and the nature of this image-guided procedure, a patient should first be seen in a clinic setting. This optimizes patient–physician rapport and allows for an appropriate discussion of risks, benefits, potential complications, outcomes, and specific details of the procedure.

In addition to risks associated with any minimally invasive procedure performed under conscious sedation (i.e., infection, bleeding, allergy to medications, damage to structures), one should include a frank discussion with the patient detailing the risks to ovarian func-tion and fertility. Based on literature reviews, there are little data on the impact of ovarian/internal iliac varices embolization on ovarian function (i.e., impact on fertility). In limited published series, and in the authors' experience, there appears to be no negative impact on the menstrual cycle or fertility [10, 19].

The patient should have a negative pregnancy test. This is a medical–legal requirement at the authors' institution.

In general, a patient is informed that should she have significant discomfort after the embolization procedure, she may be admitted to the hospital for a "short stay" primarily for pain management. In the authors' experience, post-procedure pain is significant when using sclerosing agents in the ovarian varices (as opposed to use in the internal iliac veins). (See Technique section in this chapter.) This pain can typically be managed with a short-term course of an opiate analgesic medication.

Technique

Materials

Catheters and Wires

Operator choice dictates preference. The types of catheters will depend on whether the percutaneous venous access is femoral or jugular. The jugular approach generally utilizes a multi-purpose or "hockey stick" (angled tip) configuration; whereas the femoral approach utilizes two basic shapes: a "Hopkins hook" (accentuated cobra catheter curve) for selection of the ostium of the left ovarian vein, and a reverse curve or "Simmons" shape for selection of the ostium of the right ovarian vein. The authors prefer the femoral approach with a 7 Fr sheath, a 7 Fr guiding catheter, and a 5 Fr hydrophilic catheter that may be coaxially directed.

Embolic Agents

At the authors' institution, sclerotherapy is performed as part of the embolization procedure. Although agents vary, operators may use 5% morrhuate of sodium (American Regent, Inc. Shirley, NY) plus Gelfoam® (Pharmacia & Upjohn Co, Division of Pfizer, Inc, New York, NY) (Figs. 2.6 and 2.7). Some operators use sodium tetradecyl sulfate (Bioniche Pharma USA, Lake Forest, IL) or a polymerizing glue, n-butyl-2-cyanoacrylate or butyl cyanoacrylate NBCA [11].

Coils

Depending on the size of the target vessel, coil diameter, length, shape and wire diameter (e.g., 0.035 in., 0.018 in.) vary. Operators generally use 0.035 in. diameter, 14 cm long Nester® coils (Cook Medical Inc, Bloomington, IN). The coils used for the ovarian vein trunks are generally 6, 8, 10, and 12 mm in diameter (Fig. 2.8). If the ovarian vein trunk is small in caliber, a microcatheter may be required. The authors prefer the Renegade® STC microcatheter (Boston Scientific Corp, Natick, MA) and Interlock™ coils (Boston Scientific Corp, Natick, MA).

Recent introduction of coils that create less MR imaging artifact may be more appropriate (MReye® coils, Cook Medical Inc, Bloomington, IN). The authors have limited experience with the MReye® coils.

Fig. 2.6 Photograph of Gelfoam® (Pharmacia and Upjohn Co., Pfizer Inc., New York, NY) sheet as it is being cut into small pieces. When this thick paste is used for embolization as a sclerosant, it will tend to remain in the varicosities rather than reflux into the central venous system

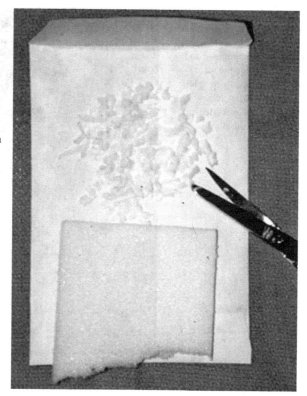

Fig. 2.7 Photograph of Gelfoam® (Pharmacia and Upjohn Co., Pfizer Inc., New York, NY) illustrating the technique of making the foam paste or "slurry." The cut pieces of Gelfoam® are placed in a 20 cm³ syringe and compressed (*vertical syringe*). The sclerosant is placed in a second 20 cm³ syringe (*horizontal syringe*)

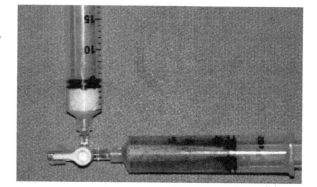

Occlusion Balloons

Use of occlusion balloons for sclerotherapy in the internal iliac system is controversial. Not all investigators agree that internal iliac veins should be evaluated and treated. Results published in the literature do suggest improved outcomes if both the ovarian and internal iliac systems are treated [10, 19]. One may use a 9 Fr occlusion balloon catheter with a 11.5 mm balloon diameter (Boston Scientific Corp, Natick, MA) for work in the internal iliac veins.

Fig. 2.8 Platinum fibered Nester® coils (Cook Medical Inc., Bloomington, IN). These coils are thrombogenic and used to occlude the main trunk(s) of incompetent left and right ovarian veins (Courtesy of Cook Medical Inc. With permission)

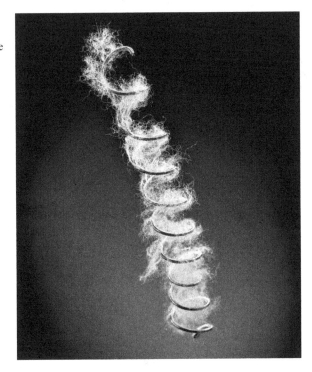

Contrast Agents

For venography, standard iodinated contrast is used. There are little data in the literature describing alternative contrast agents (e.g., carbon dioxide, gadolinium, etc.).

Procedure Start

A single dose of an antibiotic administered intravenously on the day of the procedure is utilized in some centers. Patients usually are administered intravenous sedation with short acting agents such as fentanyl and midazolam for the procedure.

The patient is placed supine, and the groins as well as the neck may be prepped and draped in the usual sterile fashion.

Step by Step

The ovarian and internal iliac veins may be approached from a jugular or femoral approach. The authors prefer the latter because of room configuration (position of monitors, etc.).

Fig. 2.9 Left ovarian venogram, same patient as in Fig. 2.5. Multiple varices are present in the left adnexal region, the pelvic floor, and adjacent to the uterus and bladder. There is also opacification of the left internal iliac venous tributaries

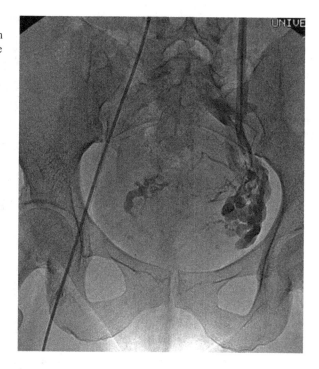

Vascular access is achieved using ultrasound guidance. A 9 Fr femoral sheath is placed. The larger 9 Fr sheath is used rather than 7 Fr to accommodate the balloon occlusion catheter used for treatment of internal iliac varices. (See earlier discussion.) A 7 Fr guiding catheter with a "Hopkins hook" shape (Cordis Johnson and Johnson, Miami Lakes, FL) is used to select the left renal vein. Once the guiding catheter tip is seated, a 5 Fr coaxially directed hydrophilic catheter is advanced over a guide wire into the ovarian vein and down into the pelvis. An ovarian venogram is performed (Fig. 2.9). After the baseline left ovarian venogram, one may mix a slurry of Gelfoam® (Pharmacia and Upjohn Co, Pfizer, Inc., New York, NY) and 5% sodium morrhuate (American Regent Laboratories, Inc., Shirley, NY).

To make this mixture, one cuts pieces of Gelfoam® (Pharmacia and Upjohn Co., Pfizer Inc., New York, NY) into small 3–4 mm pieces (Fig. 2.6). These are placed in a 20 ml syringe and compressed (Fig. 2.7). The sclerosant is placed in a second 20 ml syringe (horizontal syringe in the photograph). A three-way stopcock has been interposed between the two syringes. By pushing the syringe plungers alternately back and forth, the two materials mix together. The sclerosant soaked Gelfoam® is macerated as it passes through the hole in the barrel of the three-way stopcock. Eventually, the two mix together and become a thick paste. By partially closing the stopcock, the Gelfoam® is shredded further. This allows the paste to become more uniform in its consistency and thus easier to inject through the catheter during ovarian vein and internal iliac varices embolization.

Fig. 2.10 Completion venogram after embolization with sclerosant/Gelfoam® (Pharmacia and Upjohn Co., Pfizer Inc., New York, NY) "slurry." The left pelvic varices no longer opacify. The main left ovarian vein trunk was then occluded with embolic coils (Fig. 2.11)

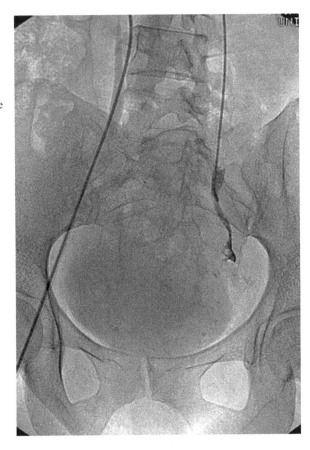

This sclerosant and Gelfoam® slurry is injected through the 5 Fr catheter. After an interval of 3–5 min (Fig. 2.10), the main left ovarian vein is occluded using coils (Figs. 2.8 and 2.11). As mentioned previously, other different sclerosing agents and glue have also been detailed in the literature.

From the inferior vena cava, the right ovarian vein is then selectively catheterized using a Simmons I or II shaped catheter (Fig. 2.12a). Some operators prefer a cobra catheter for this vein. A microcatheter is often helpful to advance access down the right ovarian vein. The microcatheter should be advanced coaxially into the right pelvic varices. After right ovarian venography, the embolization procedure is repeated using the gel foam and morrhuate slurry.

An alternative to the use of an expensive microcatheter and guidewire is the use of a Simmons-shaped 7 Fr guiding catheter and a coaxially advanced 4 or 5 Fr catheter (e.g., 5 Fr Bentson-Hanafee-Wilson 1(JB1) (Terumo Medical Corp, Somerset, NJ)). This shape is achieved by taking the Hopkins hook 7 Fr guiding catheter and heat shaping it into

Fig. 2.11 Left ovarian vein embolization with coils

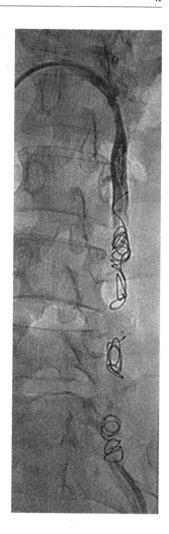

the reverse curve (i.e., Simmons) configuration. Again, after an interval of 3–5 min follow-ing slurry sclerotherapy, the main right ovarian vein is occluded using coils (Fig. 2.12b).

Given the common finding of venous communications that exist between ovarian veins and internal iliac veins, the authors feel that bilateral venography and embolization of both ovarian and internal iliac veins is required to reduce the chance of recurrence (Fig. 2.12c). It is helpful to use a balloon occlusion catheter. For this reason, a 9 Fr introducer sheath can be placed initially into the venous system. Recent introduction of occlusion balloons on a smaller diameter shaft may preclude the need for a large venous sheath size.

The authors use a 9-Fr occlusion balloon catheter with a 11.5 mm balloon diameter when inflated (Boston Scientific Corp, Natick, MA). The balloon is inflated at the anterior division

of the internal iliac vein. A venogram is performed (Fig. 2.13). The Gelfoam®-sodium morrhuate "slurry" is injected while the balloon is inflated. After a dwell time of 5–10 min, the
occlusion balloon is deflated (Fig. 2.14). In the authors' experience, use of embolic coils
should be avoided in the internal iliac veins because of the difficulty in delivering these
devices in capacious veins and the inherent risk of coil embolization to the lungs.

A staged procedure may be performed by first embolizing the right and left ovarian
varices. The patient is then allowed to recover for 3–6 weeks, and then returns later for
embolization of the pelvic internal iliac varices. This sequential approach is dictated by
practical factors such as patient personal time constraints and pain tolerance. In general,
patients experience pain after the procedure, although this pain is usually less than that
experienced by patients after arterial embolization [10, 14, 19].

If pain is severe, the patient may be admitted to the inpatient service with access to a
patient-controlled analgesia (PCA) pump (i.e., for a "short stay"). Alternatively, if enough
time is available, all four regions may be treated in one clinical setting (i.e., both ovarian
and both internal iliac veins). The authors have recently switched to a single setting embolization procedure, largely based on patient preference (avoidance of a return trip, travel,
time away from home and work, etc.).

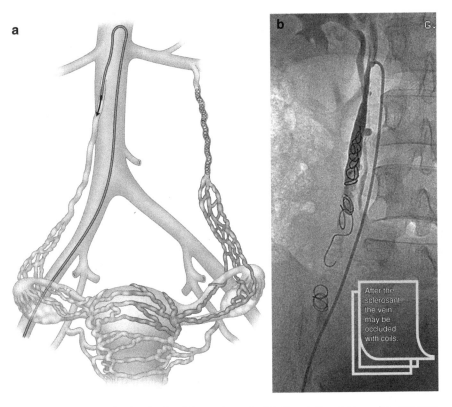

Fig. 2.12 (a) Catheter selection for the right ovarian vein. (b) Completion right ovarian venogram
after embolization of varices. (c) Catheter selection for the internal iliac vein

Fig. 2.12 (continued)

c

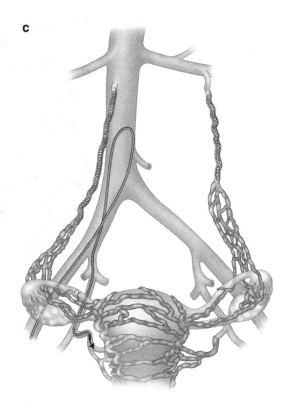

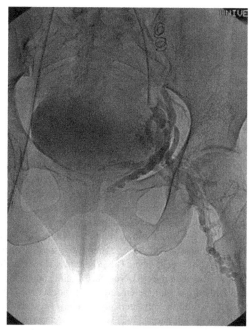

Fig. 2.13 Balloon occlusion of the internal iliac venogram from a contralateral approach. Residual varices are seen in the left pelvis. A "slurry" of sclerosant/Gelfoam® (Pharmacia and Upjohn Co., Pfizer Inc., New York, NY) was subsequently injected. The balloon was kept inflated for 10 min, then deflated

Fig. 2.14 Completed treatment of the left internal iliac varices. The varices no longer opacify

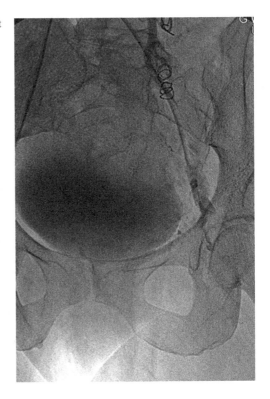

Fig. 2.15 (a–d) Fifty-year-old female with noncyclic chronic pelvic pain and rectal burning. She had a negative work up by her Gastroenterologist. She had a prior hysterectomy and bilateral salpingo-oophorectomy with no relief of symptoms. Significant past medical history included bilateral lower extremity deep venous thromboses after a motor vehicle accident 20 years ago. On physical exam, she has varices bilaterally in her thighs, buttocks, perineum, and vagina. (a) Fluoroscopic scout shows multiple calcified phleboliths in the low pelvis. (b) Left internal iliac venogram using balloon occlusion technique. Contrast refluxes from the left internal iliac vein into the left groin area and into the abnormal left lower extremity venous system. (c) Venogram performed during direct puncture of the right labia. The needle was slowly withdrawn until venous blood was aspirated. Contrast was then injected. Note the opacification of right perineal varices that were subsequently occluded with a dilute sclerosing agent (not shown). (d) Venogram of direct left labial puncture. Note reflux into the left internal iliac venous system. This communication between the left labial veins and the left internal iliac veins was occluded using the dilute sclerosing agent (not shown)

Occasionally, patients may have complex varices as a result of venous incompetence from multiple sources. Symptomatic perineal and vulvar/vaginal varices may require direct percutaneous puncture and sclerosis in addition to the transcatheter techniques described earlier (Fig. 2.15a–d).

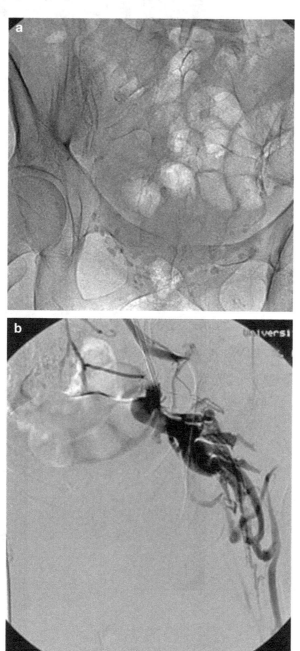

Fig. 2.15 (continued)

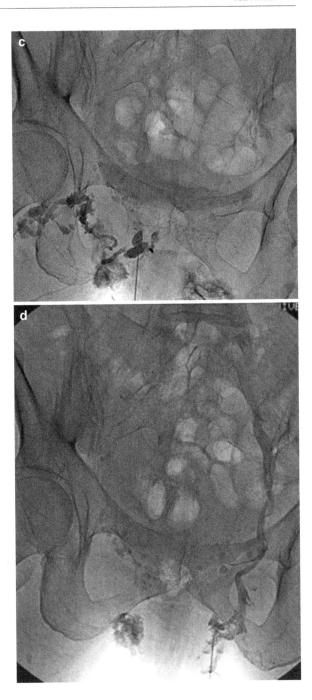

In the literature, procedural technical success rates for pelvic vein embolization have been shown to be as high as 99%.

Hints, Technical Pitfalls, and Pearls

When engaging the orifice of the ovarian vein, one may occasionally encounter vasospasm. Use of a pharmacologic vasodilator (e.g., nitroglycerine in 100 μg aliquots) injected in the ovarian vein may be useful. Alternatively, slow, direct, continuous infusion of saline into the ovarian vein orifice for several minutes may relieve venospasm. Waiting for several minutes without further wire or catheter manipulation may also result in relief of vasospasm.

If a valve in the ovarian vein prevents passage of a catheter, gentle manipulation (i.e., gentle probing with a 0.018 in. or 0.0014 in. in diameter guidewire) may prove useful. This maneuver may also be performed while the patient performs a Valsalva.

Given reports of coil embolization to the lungs during internal iliac varices embolization (early experience), the authors recommend that coils not be used in the main trunk of the internal iliac veins. Occasionally, an embolic coil may be used peripherally in the internal iliac system to close a "bridging vein" that would otherwise cause reflux of sclerosant to non-target sites (e.g., reflux of sclerosant from the internal iliac system to the saphenofemoral junction and veins of the upper thigh).

Post-Operative Care, Discharge Instructions, and Follow-up

After the procedure, access to oral, intramuscular, or intravenous pain medications may be required in the recovery room.

At discharge, patients will generally need a prescription for pain medication. At the authors' institution, the patient is also given a short course of oral antibiotics and an antiemetic. Discharge instructions and a physician contact number are also provided to the patient.

Most patients may return to normal activity within 3–5 days. Follow up in clinic in 3–6 weeks should be scheduled to assess the patient's pelvic pain and decide if further endovascular therapy is needed.

Outcomes

Previous studies have reported significant clinical improvement in 50–100% of patients undergoing embolization for PVI (PCS) [11, 14, 18–26]. In 2006, Kim et al. published the first major study of embolotherapy with both a large patient cohort ($n = 127$) and long-term follow-up (mean 45 months) [11]. From this study, 83% of patients ($n=80$, out of 97 patients with long-term follow-up) exhibited significant clinical improvement, 13% reported no significant change, and 4% experienced worse symptoms [11]. Statistically significant improvement in overall pain was noted, as well as a reduction in the following:

pain while standing, pain while lying down, dyspareunia, urinary frequency, and the number of pain medications required ($P < 0.0001$) [11].

In contrast, medical therapy has been shown to give patients relief, but the results may be short lived [27]. An extensive review of the literature for follow up of medical therapy revealed only one article with a follow-up term of 1 year – the longest documented [15]. Therefore, it is unclear if the benefits of contemporary chemical ligation for pelvic varices are truly sustained long term. Moreover, side effects of GnRH agonists and hormonal treatments – including weight gain, hot flashes, bone loss, and mood changes, which might be offset by estrogen "add-back" therapy – cannot be overlooked [27]. Further trials are needed to establish the efficacy of the GnRH/estrogen combination [27]. Even though relief from pain is not sustained in the long term with hormonal therapy, it may be most acceptable in those looking for a nonsurgical/noninterventional treatment.

Nonmedical therapy in the treatment of PCS has evolved dramatically since the 1980s. Previous studies had shown that hysterectomy with oophorectomy gave moderate relief to patients with PVI (PCS), but a recurrence rate or residual pain in 30% of patients at 1 year [17] (Fig. 2.16). Ten years ago, surgical ligation and embolization were also shown to be nearly equal in efficacy in reducing patient symptomatology for about 70% of PVI (PCS) patients treated. Experience continues to be quite limited for outcome with surgical/laparoscopic ligation of ovarian veins, with only small investigative cohorts involved [28, 29]. Moreover, surgical treatments, including hysterectomy with or without bilateral salpingo-oophorectomy and laparoscopic ligation of bilateral ovarian veins, present their own specific

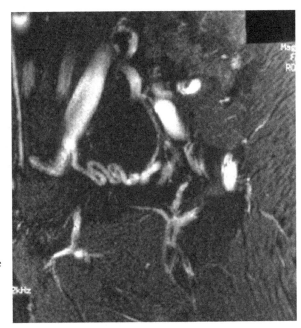

Fig. 2.16 Pelvic MRI from a woman with chronic pelvic pain who had undergone a hysterectomy. Despite this, the patient still had symptoms of pain. Pelvic varicosities arising from the iliac system are still visible

complications. Hysterectomy is associated with longer hospital stay and delayed restoration to normal daily life. Moreover, if performed with bilateral oophorectomy, it prematurely induces a menopausal state and ends the reproductive potential of a premenopausal woman. Even with laparoscopic procedures employed, 20% of the patients experience unsatisfactory results [17]. Small series of bilateral laparoscopic ligation boast absence of complications, but also acknowledge that the same may not hold in future studies with a larger sample size [30]. The procedure is also technically challenging. Multiple main trunks off the ovarian vein in as many as 40% of cases on the left and 25% of cases on the right may make laparoscopic procedures difficult, with a high potential of recurrence resulting from inadequate obliteration of all channels. In a series by Gargiulo et al. in 2003, complete remission of pain and absence of pelvic varicosities in patients who underwent surgical ligation lasted up to 12 months [28]. The authors were unsure in their conclusion whether transcatheter embolization was better, as this was not a randomized trial and patient numbers were small. Surgical management may also add the risk of abdominal and pelvic adhesion formation, ultimately increasing pain and significant patient morbidity.

Complications

Complications of embolotherapy for PVI are rare. As mentioned earlier, a few incidents of coil embolization to the pulmonary circulation during the procedure have been reported [10, 19] This rare complication may be quickly corrected by snaring and removing the coils during the procedure.

Historically, one study reported complications of treatment of PVI to include vessel perforation, non-target embolization including embolization of coils to the pulmonary circulation, and cardiac arrhythmias in 8% of patients [31]. However, in the authors' experience, reports of complications of embolotherapy are rare (less than 2%). Other investigators have reported complications less than 4% to include ovarian vein thrombophlebitis, recurrence of varices, non-target embolization of embolic material, and radiation exposure to ovaries. It is important to note that limited long-term data have thus far demonstrated no negative effects on menstrual cycle or fertility from transcatheter embolotherapy [11, 14, 19]. Kim et al. have reported that patients with PVI who underwent ovarian and pelvic varices have a more durable result in terms of reduction of their pelvic pain [11].

Also in this reported series, patients who had venous embolotherapy showed no significant change in menses, fertility, or hormone levels. Finally, a subset of patients who had previously undergone hysterectomy before embolization still achieved significant improvement based on numeric pain perception scores. Long-term results published by Kim et al. reported no major complications and also did not find any significant changes in follicle stimulating hormone (FSH), leutinizing hormone (LH), or estradiol levels. One reported topic of concern is the impact of transcatheter embolotherapy of varices on the patient's future fertility. Kim et al. reported a 50% pregnancy rate in premenopausal women who would otherwise become infertile with other medical or surgical techniques [11, 14, 19].

Summary and Conclusions

Chronic pelvic pain caused by ovarian and internal iliac varices may be managed by transcatheter techniques. Embolotherapy to include use of sclerosing agents and embolic coils is associated with a high technical and clinical success. The greatest challenge to successful outcomes is careful patient selection [32]. Complications are fortunately infrequent. Noninvasive imaging in a woman with clinical symptoms of PVI (PCS) is indicated not only to confirm the diagnosis but also to rule out other abdominal/pelvic pathology. Imaging is not completely accurate as studies are generally performed supine. Laparoscopy also is limited for reasons outlined previously. Venography is utilized with the intent to treat.

Transcatheter techniques provide a reasonable therapeutic option in the management of women with chronic pelvic pain due to ovarian and internal iliac varices.

Acknowledgment   The authors wish to express their thanks to Ms. Shundra Dinkins for her expertise in the preparation of this manuscript.

References

1. Robinson JC. Chronic pelvic pain. Curr Opin Obstet Gynecol. 1993;5:740–3.
2. Jamieson D, Steege J. The prevalence of dysmenorrhea, dyspareunia, pelvic pain, and irritable bowel syndrome in primary care practices. Obstet Gynecol. 1996;87:55–8.
3. Taylor HC. Vascular congestion and hyperemia; their effects on structure and function in the female reproductive system. Am J Obstet Gynecol. 1949;57:637–53.
4. Richet MA. Traite practique d'anatomie medico-chirurgicale. Paris: E Chemeror, Libraire Editeur; 1857.
5. Cotte G. Les troubles functionelles de l'appareil genital de la femme. Paris: Masson et Cie; 1928.
6. Ganeshan A, Upponi S, Hon LQ, Uthappa MC, Warakaulle DR, Uberoi R. Chronic pelvic pain due to pelvic congestion syndrome: the role of diagnostic and interventional radiology. Cardiovasc Intervent Radiol. 2007;30(6):1105–11.
7. Stones RW. Pelvic vascular congestion – half a century later. Clin Obstet Gynecol. 2003;46:831–6.
8. Giacchetto C, Catizone F, Cotroneo GB, et al. Radiologic anatomy of the genital venous system in female patients with varicocele. Surg Gynecol Obstet. 1989;169:403–7.
9. Lefevre H. Broad ligament varicocele. Acta Obstet Gynecol Scand. 1964;41:122–3.
10. Scultetus AH, Villavicencio JL, Gillespie DL. The nutcracker syndrome: its role in the pelvic venous disorders. J Vasc Surg. 2001;34:812–9.
11. Kim HS, Malhotra AD, Rowe PC, Lee JM, Venbrux AC. Embolotherapy for pelvic congestion syndrome: long-term results. J Vasc Interv Radiol. 2006;17(2 Pt 1):289–97.
12. Park SJ, Lim JW, Ko YT, Lee DH, Yoon Y, Oh JH, et al. Diagnosis of pelvic congestion syndrome using transabdominal and transvaginal sonography. AJR Am J Roentgenol. 2004;182:683–8.
13. Beard RW, Highman JH, Pearce S, et al. Diagnosis of pelvic varicosities in women with chronic pelvic pain. Lancet. 1984;2(8409):946–949.
14. Ignacio EA, Dua R, Sarin S, Harper AS, Yim D, Mathur V, et al. Pelvic congestion syndrome: diagnosis and treatment. Women's issues in interventional radiology. Semin Intervent Radiol. 2008;25:361–8.

15. Soysal ME, Soysal S, Vicdan K, Ozer S. A randomized controlled trial of goserelin and medroxyprogesterone acetate in the treatment of pelvic congestion. Hum Reprod. 2001;16(5):931–9.
16. Beard RW, Kennedy RG, Gangar KF, et al. Bilateral oophorectomy and hysterectomy in the treatment of intractable pelvic pain associated with pelvic congestion. Br J Obstet Gynaecol. 1991;98:988–92.
17. Carter J. Surgical treatment for chronic pelvic pain. JSLS. 1998;2:129–39.
18. Edwards RD, Robertson IR, MacLean AB, et al. Case report: pelvic pain syndrome – successful treatment of a case by ovarian vein embolization. Clin Radiol. 1993;47:429–31.
19. Venbrux AC, Chang AH, Kim HS, et al. Pelvic congestion syndrome (pelvic venous incompetence): impact of ovarian and internal iliac vein embolotherapy on menstrual cycle and chronic pelvic pain. J Vasc Interv Radiol. 2002;13:171–8.
20. Sichlau MJ, Yao JS, Vogelzang RL. Transcatheter embolotherapy for the treatment of pelvic congestion syndrome. Obstet Gynecol. 1994;83:892–6.
21. Tarazov PG, Prozorovskij KV, Ryzhkov VK. Pelvic pain syndrome caused by ovarian varices: treatment by transcatheter embolization. Acta Radiol. 1997;38:1023–5.
22. Capasso P, Simons C, Trotteur G, et al. Treatment of symptomatic pelvic varices by ovarian vein embolization. Cardiovasc Intervent Radiol. 1997;20:107–11.
23. Cordts PR, Eclavea A, Buckley PJ, et al. Pelvic congestion syndrome: early clinical results after transcatheter ovarian vein embolization. J Vasc Surg. 1998;28:862–8.
24. Maleux G, Stockx L, Wilms G, et al. Ovarian vein embolization for the treatment of pelvic congestion syndrome: long-term technical and clinical results. J Vasc Interv Radiol. 2000;11:859–64.
25. Pieri S, Agresti P, Morucci M, et al. Percutaneous treatment of pelvic congestion syndrome. Radiol Med (Torino). 2003;105:76–82.
26. Bachar GN, Belenky A, Greif F, et al. Initial experience with ovarian vein embolization for the treatment of chronic pelvic pain syndrome. Isr Med Assoc J. 2003;12:843–6.
27. Stone W, Cheong YC, Howard FM. Interventions for treating chronic pain in women. Cochrane Database Syst Rev 2005; (2): CD000387. DOI:10.1002/14651858.
28. Gargiulo T, Mais V, Brokaj L, Cossu E, Melis GB. Bilateral laparoscopic transperitoneal ligation of ovarian veins for treatment of pelvic congestion syndrome. J Am Assoc Gynecol Laparosc. 2003;10(4):501–4.
29. Chung M-H, Huh C-Y. Comparison of treatments for pelvic congestion syndrome. Tohoku J Exp Med. 2003;201:131–8.
30. Takeuchi K, Mochizuki M, Kitagaki S. Laparoscopic varicocele ligation for pelvic congestion syndrome. Int J Gynaecol Obstet. 1996;55:177–8.
31. Coakley FV, Varghese SL, Hricak H. CT and MRI of pelvic varices in women. J Comput Assist Tomogr. 1999;23:429–34.
32. Millward S, Black C, Thorpe K, Venbrux A, et al. Research reporting standards for endovascular treatment of pelvic venous insufficiency. J Vasc Interv Radiol. 2010;21:796–803.

Part II

Fallopian Tube Interventions

Fallopian Tube Recanalization

3

Elizabeth Ann Ignacio, Taara Sultaana Hassan, John C. Lipman, and Farhang Adabi

Introduction

With infertility prevalence data ranging from 7% to 20% in the United States, reproductive assistance methods are an important medical concern [1, 2]. In working up the infertile couple, practitioners must exclude anatomic causes. When proper work-up and imaging reveal a proximal fallopian tube occlusion, recanalization is a reasonably straightforward and low-risk procedure that can be beneficial to these patients.

When proper work-up and imaging reveal a proximal fallopian tube occlusion, recanalization is a reasonably straightforward and low-risk procedure that can be beneficial to these patients.

Due to its minimally invasive approach and low risks, selective salpingography with fallopian tube recanalization (FTR) has emerged as a nonsurgical treatment option for women with infertility secondary to proximal tubal obstruction [3–7]. Reported success rates in achieving tubal patency have ranged from 75% to 95%, with subsequent successful intrauterine pregnancy rates averaging between 30% and 40% [3, 5, 6, 8, 9]. It is the hope of the authors that Interventionalists will familiarize themselves with this technique so as to offer patients a relatively simple, cost-effective method to treat infertility.

Pathophysiology

The prevalence of cellular debris in women with proximal tubal obstruction has been reported as high as 77% [10]. Reports have shown mucous plugs and proteinaceous material being the etiology in the majority of proximal tubal obstructions [11]. Other etiologies include fibrosis, scarring (often secondary to pelvic inflammatory disease), adhesions of tubal ligation reversal surgery, salpingitis isthmica nodosa, and intermittent tubal spasm [3, 12, 13].

E.A. Ignacio (✉)
Department of Radiology, Division of Interventional Radiology,
The George Washington University Medical Center, Washington, DC, USA
e-mail: eaignaciomd@gmail.com

E.A. Ignacio and A.C. Venbrux (eds.), *Women's Health in Interventional Radiology*,
DOI 10.1007/978-1-4419-5876-1_3, © Springer Science+Business Media, LLC 2012

Fig. 3.1 Hydrosalpinx. Fallopian tube obstruction. There is no free spillage of contrast into the pelvis

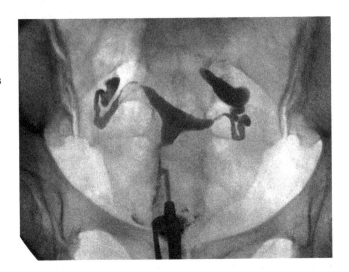

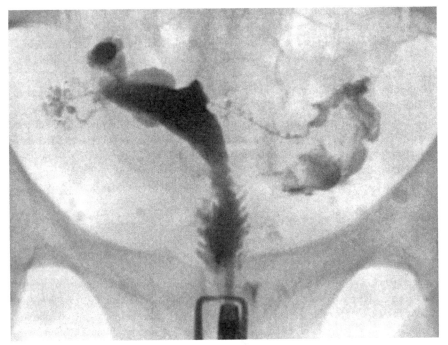

Fig. 3.2 Salpingitis isthmica nodosum

Fibrosis and scarring are frequent causes of proximal tubal obstruction. Often, this is secondary to pelvic inflammatory disease, commonly Chlamydia trachomatis. Salpingitis may be associated with endometritis and oophoritis (Fig. 3.1). These infectious etiologies as well as septic abortion may cause severe and/or chronic inflammation rendering the fallopian tubes dysfunctional due to fibrosis, adhesions, or ciliary damage [12].

Adhesions secondary to reversal of prior tubal ligation are also a cause of proximal tubal obstruction. Reports have shown that patency is achieved in approximately 68% of patients. Of those reversals, subsequent successful intrauterine pregnancies are associated with a shorter timeframe between the procedure and conception [14].

Salpingitis Isthmica Nodosa (SIN) is a relatively rare yet well-known cause of tubal obstruction. It is characterized as pathologic diverticula of the fallopian tube epithelium often accompanied by nodular hyperplasia (Fig. 3.2). Review of literature found its incidence in healthy, fertile women to range from 0.6% to 11% [15]. However, it is more common in the setting of ectopic pregnancy, with incidence reports between 7% and 25% (versus an average of 3% for other etiologies) [13, 15].

Current treatment options available to patients with proximal tubal obstruction include surgery such as salpingolysis and tuboplasty, hysteroscopic tubal cannulation, selective salpingography with fallopian tube recanalization, and in-vitro fertilization (IVF) [5, 7]. In the absence of underlying tubal pathology, fallopian tube catheterization has the potential to be therapeutic by dislodging the obstructive debris [16].

Clinical Manifestations

Infertility is generally defined as the inability to conceive after 12 months of unprotected sexual intercourse [17, 18]. While this is the main clinical manifestation of patients seeking treatment of proximal fallopian tube occlusion, primary infertility has a long list of possible causes, and the additional clinical manifestations may be widely varied depending on the specific etiologies.

Anatomy

The Female Reproductive Organs

The female reproductive tract includes: the vagina, the cervix, the uterus, the fallopian tubes, and the ovaries (Fig. 3.3a).

The vagina, on average, is an 8-cm tubular structure that lies inferior to the urethra and bladder fundus and superior to anal canal and rectum. Ordinarily, it extends dorso-cephalically, terminating at the vaginal portion of cervix where it forms anterior and posterior recesses (i.e., anterior and posterior fornix). The posterior fornix is usually greater in size. The vaginal mucosa contains variable-sized rugae covered by stratified squamous epithelium giving it its undulating appearance. The submucosa contains large, anastomosing veins.

The cervix is the distal, conical segment of the uterus that projects into the vagina between the anterior and posterior fornices forming the external os. It is constricted at the start and terminus with a more dilated middle segment. The cervical mucosa is distinct from the uterine cavity with a papillar, viscous characteristic.

The body of a non-gravid uterus is a flattened, thick-walled, triangular organ, lying superio-posteriorly to the bladder. While its actual size will depend on the age

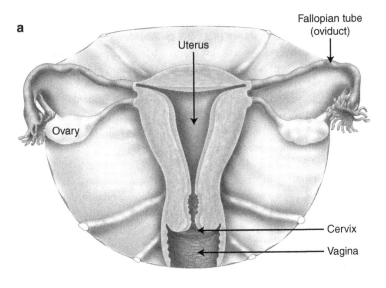

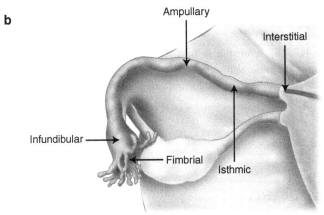

Fig. 3.3 (a) The female pelvis. (b) The fallopian tube

and individual anatomy of the patient, the average nulliparous adult uterus is approximately 8 cm long, 5 cm wide, and 2.5 cm thick [19]. The upper portion, or the base, lies between the openings of the fallopian tubes, one on either side; and the lower portion, the apex, communicates with the vagina via the cervix. Depending on the phase in the menstrual cycle, the mucosa can be relatively pale and smooth or hyperremic and rugal in appearance.

The ovaries are the female gonads and also have endocrine function as well. Each ovary is approximately 4 cm and is held in place medially by the ovarian ligament and the suspensory ligament of the ovary. Part of the broad ligament covers the ovary and is called the mesovarium.

The fallopian tubes provide passage of the ovum from the ovary toward the uterus. There is one fallopian tube on each side that extends laterally from the superior angles of the uterus. The tube is in the upper part of the broad ligament between the round and utero-ovarian ligaments. Each tube is approximately 10 cm long and consists of three external segments beyond the interstitial intramural portion of the uterus (Fig. 3.3b):

1. Isthmus: constricted, proximal third (approximately 1–2 mm in diameter)
2. Ampulla: middle, dilated third (approximately 5–10 mm in diameter)
3. Infundibulum: terminal third abutting the ovary.

The fallopian tube mucosa is continuous with the uterus and gradually becomes columnar and ciliated [20]. Cilia are most prominent in the fimbriated infundibulum. At the infundibulum, the fallopian tubes turn downward over the medial surface of the ovary. The irregular fimbriae come in close apposition to the ovary.

It is peristaltic contraction of smooth muscle fibers in the fallopian tube wall, ciliary activity, and the rich tubal fluid secreted by the epithelium that promote transport of the sperm and egg ultimately for fertilization.

Imaging

The Hysterosalpingogram (HSG)

Historically, laparoscopy with chromotubation has been the gold standard for assessing patency of fallopian tubes [21]. This procedure involves using laparoscopy to visualize the course of dye injected through the vagina into the uterus and fallopian tubes. However, due to a less invasive nature and no need for anesthesia, most clinicians utilize the hysterosalpingogram (HSG) to assess tubal factors of infertility [22].

Hysterosalpingograms (HSG) have long been used as a safe and effective method in the initial evaluation of an infertile woman [7]. It enables the physician to identify any abnormalities in the shape and size of the uterus and/or fallopian tubes that may be the cause of infertility [23]. The American Society of Reproductive Medicine has recommended that an HSG be a part of an optimal work-up of the infertile female [23].

In particular, evaluating tubal patency is a critical component of infertility diagnosis as HSGs have identified proximal fallopian tube obstruction in approximately 15–20% of cases [3–5].

In an HSG, contrast dye is injected into the cervical canal, and fluoroscopic images are obtained. A normal result shows filling of the uterine cavity, which is normally triangular shaped with a mildly concave fundus. As the contrast enters the isthmus of the fallopian tubes bilaterally, it should appear thin and threadlike. Progressing to the dilated ampulla, the contrast expands, outlining rugal folds until it spills with fanning into the peritoneal cavity (Fig. 3.4). Abnormalities seen may include filling defects, excessive tortuosity, single fallopian tubes, and/or spillage along the course of the fallopian tube [24].

Fig. 3.4 Hystero-salpingogram. Normal contrast filling of uterine cavity, fallopian tubes, and spillage to peritoneal cavity

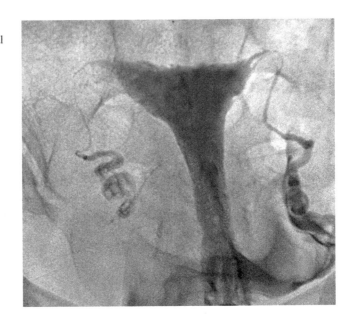

Patient Encounter

Indications and Contraindications

Documented infertility for 12 months of unprotected sex is the only indication for this procedure.

Contraindications for fallopian tube recanalization are also straightforward. The presence of an active pelvic infection is an absolute contraindication. If the patient has a history of recent pelvic infection, it is imperative to verify complete resolution before proceeding further. Other important contraindications include menstruation, pregnancy, recent pelvic procedure such as dilatation and curettage, severe cardiac or renal disease, uterine malignancy, i.e., endometrial carcinoma, and sensitivity to contrast media.

Consult, Consent, and Preparation

A consult visit with the patient and family pre-procedure is optimal for planning, proper patient preparation, and setting of expectations. Certainly, the male partner should also undergo a complete fertility work-up, and all abnormalities should be corrected even if the fallopian tube procedure is an option. Discussion of the procedure should touch on common questions of pain, bleeding, and infection. While pain does occur, it is usually limited in duration and rarely requires medication beyond standard over the counter analgesics. Women may have some spotting post procedure, but significant bleeding after recanalization is rare. Infection is a strict contraindication. This risk should be carefully reviewed with respect to the patient's past medical history, and prophylactic antibiotics should be prescribed. The risk for ectopic pregnancy exists, is 3%, and must be disclosed to all potential patients. This discussion should be tempered by the patient's preexisiting history of tubal pregnancy. (See sections in this chapter on Outcomes and Complications.) Finally, it is very important and helpful for the patient and family to understand the rate of conception following fallopian tube recanalization, which has been reported close to 40% [7].

Patients with infertility secondary to tubal occlusion are usually referred from fertility specialists to the Interventional Radiologist for fallopian tube recanalization. Most patients have already gone through the diagnostic work-up, and tubal obstruction has been documented by a previous hysterosalpingogram (HSG). A review of the pertinent images with the patient and partner is helpful.

Timing of the procedure is essential to safety and overall success. To reduce the risk of iatrogenic endometriosis, the procedure should be performed at a time when the patient is not menstruating. The patient is also advised to abstain from sexual intercourse in the days after her menses and prior to the procedure, to ensure that she is not pregnant during the procedure. This is very important. Generally, day 7–10 in a 28-day cycle is appropriate for the procedure, i.e., after cessation of menstrual flow and before ovulation when the endometrium is stable.

A negative serum pregnancy test may be acquired on the day of the procedure. Given the use of fluoroscopy, this is a medical–legal requirement at the authors' institution.

In the absence of any other preexisting medical condition, no other labs may be required. Some operators may desire a complete pelvic exam with cervical swab as well as preoperative white blood cell count in order to document the absence of a smoldering pelvic infection.

With regards to antibiotics, the American College of Obstetricians and Gynecologists recommends no prophylaxis for patients without history of pelvic infection undergoing simple hysterosalpingography. However, if salpingography demonstrates dilated fallopian tubes, antibiotic prophylaxis should be given to reduce the incidence of post-HSG pelvic inflammatory disease (PID) [25]. For transcervical procedures, prophylaxis may be considered in those patients with a history of PID or previously documented tubal abnormality or damage.

At the authors' institution, patients who are preoperative for recanalization are routinely prophylaxed. Although antibiotic regimens vary, oral doxycycline therapy is generally prescribed. One accepted regimen is doxycycline 100 mg, one tablet by mouth twice a day beginning 2 days before the procedure, the day of the procedure, and then for 2 days after the procedure (10 tablets dispensed).

Technique

Materials

Vaginal Speculum

Disposable plastic vaginal specula are available in sizes small, medium, and large. A light source is needed, and there are some disposable specula with an attached LED light that are especially helpful for direct visualization of the cervix. A metallic speculum may be used; however, metal is radiopaque and limits visualization of the vaginal vault under fluoroscopy.

Transcervical Catheters

There are many catheter choices for uterine access. Like many interventional radiology tools, these catheter tips may have different shapes and vary in stiffness in order to assist transcervical placement.

Some of the authors at our institution use the Thurmond-Rosch Movable Cup Hysterocath® (Cook Medical Inc, Bloomington, IN). This is a 28-Fr catheter, 24 cm long with an acorn-shaped tip to engage the external cervical os. Note that this catheter never traverses the cervix into the uterine cavity, but the large caliber allows for the coaxial placement of tools without interference. The small concentric plastic cup comes in three sizes, and is advanced down the shaft in order to fit closely over the cervix. This cervical cup has a microtube that can be hooked up to wall suction for gentle adherence to the cervix during the procedure. Placement of this sheath-like device decreases repeated dilatation across the cervix, and prevents access from being lost during the subsequent wire and catheter manipulations (Fig. 3.5).

Another author preference is the Cook Intrauterine Access balloon catheter (Cook Medical Inc, Bloomington, IN). This catheter is 9 Fr in size (3 mm outer diameter) and does traverse the cervical os. A sidearm is present in order to flush or inject contrast during the entire procedure. Further, the proximal balloon is inflated through a separate port to maintain access, and it does not inhibit manipulations at the distal catheter tip (Fig. 3.6a, b).

Catheters and Wires

Any variation of a hockey stick-shaped directional 5 Fr catheter may be used, depending on the operator's preference. A soft 035 wire is needed as well. The authors prefer the 5.5 Fr 50 cm catheter and 035 "J" tip wire of the Fallopian Tube Catheterization Set (Cook Medical Inc, Bloomington, IN).

A separate 5 or 6 Fr balloon catheter is another option that some operators prefer for the hysterosalpingogram alone.

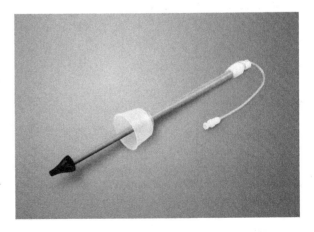

Fig. 3.5 Thurmond Hysterocath® (Cook Medical Inc, Bloomington, IN), acorn tip, cervical cup (Courtesy of Cook Medical, Inc. With permission)

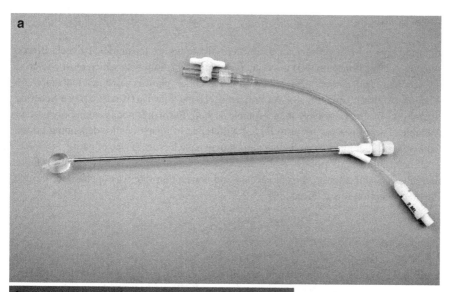

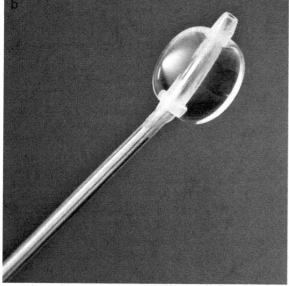

Fig. 3.6 (a) Cook Intrauterine Access balloon catheter (Cook Medical Inc, Bloomington, IN, sideport for flushing or injections. (b) Proximal balloon (Courtesy of Cook Medical, Inc. With permission)

A 3 Fr or smaller catheter and soft 0.018 wire are typically used for the recanalization. The authors use the 3 Fr 65 cm catheter in the Cook Fallopian Tube Catheterization Set (Cook Medical Inc, Bloomington, IN) and the included 0.018 wire.

Other 0.018 wire options that may be helpful include a hydrophilic 0.018 wire and also a straight 0.018 wire (please see Step by Step discussion in the section that follows). A torque device can also be used.

Contrast Agents

Iodinated contrast is necessary for the hysterosalpingogram. Iopamidol (Isovue®, Bracco Imaging, S.P.A., Princeton, NJ) is a nonionic contrast medium with which most operators are familiar. The authors use iopamidol-300. Other choices such as iodixanol-320 (Visipaque®, Bracco Imaging, S.P.A., Princeton, NJ) and iotrolan (Isovist®, Bayer Schering Pharma AG Berlin, Germany) are acceptable as well. Iotrolan is not as commonly used or available. There does not seem to be any difference in image quality depending on the contrast agent, but iotrolan nonionic contrast may have less incidence of pain.

Of note, Pinto et al. reported that with the use of an oil-based contrast agent for fallopian tube recanalization, technical success and conception rate was unchanged, but the time to conception was reduced [26].

Cervical Os Finder, Cervical Dilator, Uterine Sound

A cervical os finder is a tapered and smooth tool, ideal for seeking the cervical os. This instrument is not required for transcervical access, but it can be helpful to gently open the cervical os.

A cervical dilator may also assist transcervical access. Dilators can vary in size from 3/4 mm to 25/26 mm. The cervical dilator may be particularly helpful for patients with cervical stenosis.

A uterine sound is a tool used to measure uterine depth and the distance between the cervical os and uterine fundus, but this can also be helpful in patients who have cervical stenosis. The proximal portion of the uterine sound may be 3.9 mm in diameter, tapering to 2.5 mm.

Disposable cervical os finders, dilators, and uterine sounds are commercially available.

Procedure Start

This procedure can be performed in the standard Interventional Radiology suite with fluoroscopy available. The patient lies supine with the lower extremities in the open lithotomy position, similar to that for a pelvic examination. The patient's knees may be flexed laterally (frog leg), and/or one may use surgical stirrups for support depending on the patient's comfort (Fig. 3.7a).

Intravenous sedation is optional and, once achieved, the perineum may be prepped. The perineum can be prepped with povidone–iodine scrub (Purdue Products, Stamford, CT), or even a baby shampoo/mild detergent. The area is then covered with sterile blue towels and a paper drape in the usual fashion.

Step by Step

The procedure begins with a hysterosalpingogram. A bivalved speculum is inserted into the vagina and locked in place for the procedure (Fig. 3.7a, b).

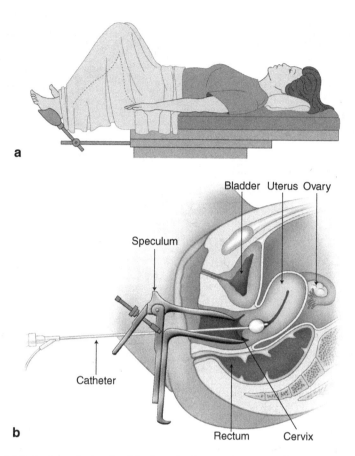

Fig. 3.7 (a) Patient positioning for fallopian tube intervention. (b) Placement of speculum and access catheter

The technique for hysterosalpingogram has been well documented. Many operators prefer to use a balloon catheter placed transcervically, with the balloon inflated at the uterine isthmus. Care should be taken that the balloon not be inflated to the cervical isthmus where it frequently causes significant patient discomfort [27]. Some authors oppose the use of an intrauterine balloon when further manipulations are planned, i.e., recanalization, since the balloon can interfere with visualization and movement of the catheters [10, 28]. In preparation for recanalization, a transcervical sheath device is helpful to maintain access and can be placed over a J tip wire. All transcervical tools should be sized appropriately for the cervical os, the internal diameter of which may be approximately 4–8 mm. Excessive cervical stretching can give non-sedated patients significant discomfort.

While some operators might use a cervical tenaculum for additional traction, it is rarely required, in the authors' experience. Applying gentle movement to the cervical tenaculum can bring the anteverted uterus into a more favorable angle for visualization of the cornua. The disadvantage of a tenaculum is that it gives the patient more pain and cervical bleeding.

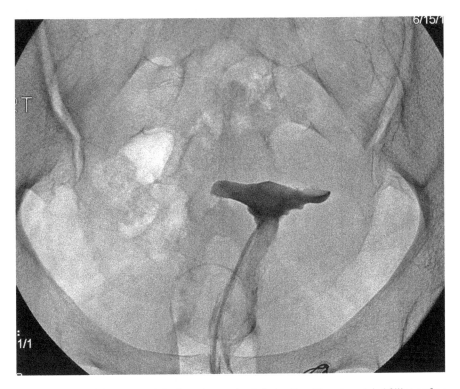

Fig. 3.8 Hysterosalpingogram. Fallopian tube proximal obstruction. There is no tubal filling or free spillage of contrast into the pelvis

Whether a sheath is used or not, a wire and catheter may be used for the intrauterine contrast injection, i.e., hysterosalpingogram. The system may be advanced under fluoroscopy, allowing for accurate centering, as tools may buckle with inadvertent placement in the vaginal fornix. When exchanging catheters and wires, care should be taken to avoid air in the uterus. Such air, when injected with contrast into the endometrial cavity, may create an artifact of polypoid filling defects during imaging.

Complete opacification of the uterus may require 10–20 ml of contrast (Fig. 3.8). These images are reviewed for the presence of mass(es) such as fibroids and/or anatomic variation, as well as normal spillage of contrast out the fallopian tubes. (See also the previous discussion on normal pelvic anatomy.) Often, a previously documented occlusion may become patent with simple salpingography alone, as the gentle contrast injection may be enough to flush out obstructive debris. In the absence of spillage, however, an obstruction is presumed, which can be secondary to various etiologies. (See Pathophysiology section in this chapter.)

For recanalization of the obstructed fallopian tube, one may readvance the J guidewire with the guiding catheter. This guidewire and catheter are directed toward the isthmus on the occluded side. The guidewire is removed. While guide catheter angulation is maintained, one can then advance a 3 Fr or smaller microcatheter coaxially through the initial guiding catheter, as the normal caliber of the fallopian tube is about 1–3 mm in diameter. The microcatheter is directed to the cornua or interstitial segment of the fallopian tube.

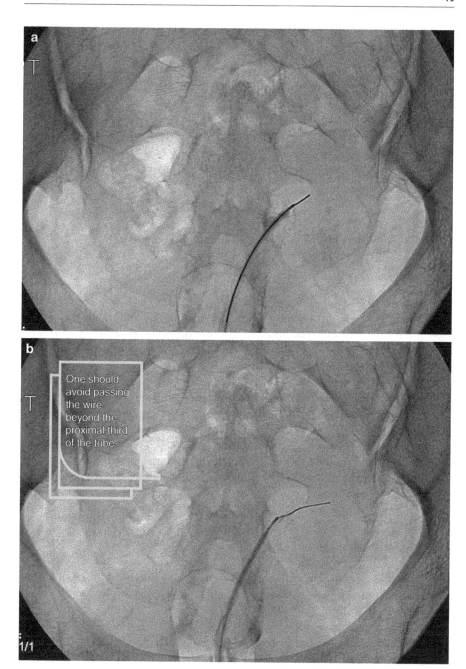

Fig. 3.9 (**a**) Catheter and wire advanced through proximal fallopian tube. (**b**) Recanalization

With gentle probing, the simple passage of a soft 0.018 wire and microcatheter through this area may open up the blockage, pushing any cellular debris distally (Fig. 3.9a). When the fallopian tube is engaged with the 0.018 wire, one should not advance the tip into the

Fig. 3.10 Normal filling. The catheter is at the left fallopian tube. Free spillage of contrast into the pelvis following recanalization

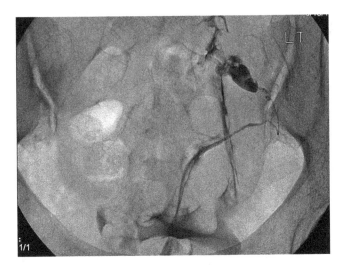

tube lumen too far. The fallopian tube is a thin relatively fragile conduit, and most operators caution against wire advancement beyond the proximal third of the tube (Fig. 3.9b). There is a risk that the wire may penetrate the mucosa, analogous to raising a vascular intimal flap. The 0.018 wire should make a gentle curve once it enters the tube lumen. It should not buckle or form a "J." A hydrophilic-coated 0.018 wire with an angled tip is sometimes useful. Alternatively, a straight-tipped 0.018 wire may allow the operator to "customize" or create the needed angulation for the wire tip. A torque device can be helpful for negotiating a tortuous proximal fallopian tube course.

Contrast can be injected to evaluate the progress of recanalization. Technical success is achieved when the fallopian tube is fully opacified, and there is contrast spillage into the pelvis (Fig. 3.10).

At the end of the recanalization procedure, the guiding catheter is taken out, and the speculum is removed.

Hints, Technical Pitfalls, and Pearls

The presence of cervical stenosis is sometimes challenging for operators. The use of a cervical dilator or also a uterine sound may be helpful. Also, one may place a transcervical catheter that is more firm.

Occasionally, recanalization of a proximal occlusion will uncover a more distal occlusion. However, these distal occlusions are more likely secondary to pelvic peritoneal processes like post-inflammatory adhesions. Scarring and adhesions are outside the tube lumen and therefore not accessible for endoluminal therapy.

In women who have had previous surgical ligation and then reversal, persistent fallopian tube occlusion may exist beyond the most proximal portion of the fallopian tube.

While this is likely a mechanical problem not necessarily amenable to recanalization therapy, some operators have had anecdotal reports of success.

Postoperative Care, Discharge Instructions, and Follow-Up

Post-procedure, the patient is recovered from any sedation. Patients are then discharged to home the same day. Discharge instructions vary for institutions. Patients are encouraged to resume normal sexual activity the next day or a few days later, depending on the level of pain and/or bleeding/spotting.

When a couple is still unable to conceive within 6 months after a successful fallopian tube recanalization, there may be consideration for a repeat hysterosalpingogram in order to evaluate for reocclusion. Repeat recanalization can also be performed at that time.

Outcomes

A high rate of technical success in fallopian tube recanalization (>95%) has been achieved as evinced by many interventional radiology authors ([29, 30, 31]), including the pioneering work of Thurmond et al. Technical outcomes may be reviewed and further qualified with respect to factors such as the presence of preexisting tubal disease and the use of specific technical steps, as selective salpingography alone versus tubal recanalization. Results and reocclusion rates may also have prognostic value for the management of infertile patients. Ultimately, the rate of conception in patients is most important for assessing the clinical effectiveness of recanalization therapy.

In a large retrospective series of 1006 patients, Li et al. reported a recanalization success rate of 87.9% [32]. Interestingly, of the tubal occlusion group, 35.4% were treated with selective salpingography alone, while 64.6% underwent fallopian tube recanalization. The postoperative pregnancy rate was 39.9% in this group. Of patients with incomplete tubal occlusion, the pregnancy rate was higher – 53.6%, 45.7%, and 26.8% – depending on the degree of occlusion categorized as mild, moderate, and severe.

Differing reports on technical success and pregnancy rates may definitely be attributed to differences in patient selection and the presence of significant preexisting tubal disease. In an unrestricted patient population, Hovsepian et al. performed 42 fallopian tube procedures [33]. Recanalization success was achieved in 71% of occlusions in the presence of considerable tubal pathology, and the conception rate was 33%. Despite a lower rate of technical success and resulting pregnancy compared to other studies, the report does show that favorable rates can be achieved from recanalization procedures even with a high prevalence of tubal disease.

While fallopian tube recanalization has been shown to be a safe and effective method for the treatment of tubal obstruction, it may also have a new role of prognostic value in the management of infertility. In a review by Papaioannou et al., data for the measurement of tubal perfusion pressures at selective salpingography and tubal catheterization

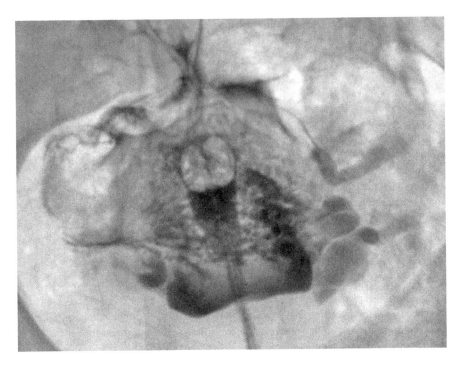

Fig. 3.11 Venous intravasation and hydrosalpinx

with subsequent classification of infertility are presented [34, 35]. This classification may correlate to the possibility of spontaneous fertility, conferring a prognostic profile for this procedure in the fertility work-up.

Complications

Selective salpingography and/or fallopian tube recanalization is a relatively simple procedure with an extremely low rate of complications and adverse clinical events.

Patients may expect some pelvic pain and cramping after the procedure. This may be secondary to the contrast distension of the uterus, a condition occasionally described as hypogastric colic. Pain may also arise from the peritoneal irritation of contrast spillage. Usually, postoperative pain is transient and may require minimal, over the counter analgesics.

Venous intravasation is an inadvertent injection of contrast through the endometrium with resultant filling of pelvic veins and lymphatics. Under fluoroscopy, one sees multiple thin lines forming a reticular pattern that washes out when injection is discontinued. This usually does not cause any adverse clinical affect [29]. Risk for intravasation is higher when the endometrium is unstable, as in menstruation or recent curretage (Fig. 3.11).

In patients with known tubal obstruction, the risk of ectopic pregnancy following recanalization exists, but this may depend on the presence of certain factors. Post-recanalization procedure, Li et al. reported a 2.7% ectopic pregnancy rate in the patient group with complete occlusions [32]. In the incomplete tubal occlusion group, the ectopic pregnancy rate was less at 1.4%. Similar rates have been reported by other authors such as Thurmond, who stated that the incidence of tubal pregnancy in a normal appearing fallopian tube following recanalization may not be any higher than that of the normal population [7, 36]. Conversely, ectopic pregnancy appears more likely in patients who have preexisting tubular pathology such as peritubal adhesions or a history of tubal surgery. In the study by Hovsepian et al. involving 37 patients, there were three tubal pregnancies in patients post recanalization, of which all three patients had had a previous history of ectopic pregnancy. Thus, the occurrence of tubal pregnancy following recanalization, although temporally related, may reflect the preexisting state of the fallopian tube before catheterization.

The risk for partial tubal perforation exists but has not been shown to have any adverse clinical events. Complete through and through perforation of the fallopian tube may manifest as contrast extravasation into the peritoneal cavity. No adverse sequelae have been reported [36].

With proper patient screening and preoperative antibiotic prophylaxis, other postoperative complications such as infection, peritonitis, and endometritis after fallopian tube recanalization are rare.

Overall, the clinical benefits of fallopian tube recanalization, coupled with the comparatively low cost and time investment of this procedure, outweigh the risks. This procedure remains an effective viable option for couples with infertility issues.

Summary and Conclusions

Fallopian tube recanalization has proven to be a worthwhile procedure for women with infertility secondary to fallopian tube disease. The technique and clinical work for fallopian tube recanalization are evenly accessible to the Interventional Radiologist, and this treatment option may offer a profound benefit for properly selected infertile patients. For operators, the catheter manipulations are straightforward, and the technical success is high. While there is risk for serious complication such as ectopic pregnancy, the rates are quite low. A simple elegant procedure, fallopian tube recanalization is safe and effective for women with infertility secondary to fallopian tube occlusion and an essential tool for physicians in their therapeutic armamentarium for infertility.

References

1. National Survey of Family Growth: Infertility. Centers for Disease Control. Atlanta, GA. December 2002. http://www.cdc.gov/nchs/nsfg/abc_list_i.htm#infertility. Accessed July 15, 2010.
2. Boivin J, Bunting L, Collins JA, Nygren KG. International estimates of infertility prevalence and treatment-seeking: potential need and demand for infertility medical care. Hum Reprod. 2007;22(6):1506–12.
3. Thurmond AS. Selective salpingography and fallopian tube recanalization. AJR Am J Roentgenol. 1991;156(1):33–8.

4. Novy MJ, Thurmond AS, Patton P, Uchida BT, Rosch J. Diagnosis of cornual obstruction by transcervical fallopian tube cannulation. Fertil Steril. 1988;50(3):434–40.
5. Verma A, Krarup K, Donuru A. Selective salpingography and fallopian tube catheterisation by guidewire. J Obstet Gynaecol. 2009;29(4):315–7.
6. Hayashi M, Hoshimoto K, Ohkura T. Successful conception following fallopian tube recanalization in infertile patients with a unilateral proximally occluded tube and a contralateral patent tube. Hum Reprod. 2003;18(1):96–9.
7. Thurmond AS, Thurmond AS, Machan L, Maubon AJ, et al. A review of selective salpingography and fallopian tube recanalization. Radiographics. 2000;20:1759–68.
8. Al-Jaroudi D, Herba MJ, Tulandi T. Reproductive performance after selective tubal catheterization. J Minim Invasive Gynecol. 2005;12(2):150–2.
9. Lang EK, Dunaway Jr HE. Efficacy of salpingography and transcervical recanalization in diagnosis, categorization, and treatment of fallopian tube obstruction. Cardiovasc Intervent Radiol. 2000;23(6):417–22.
10. Thurmond AS. Selective salpingography and fallopian tube recanalization. AJR Am J Roentgenol. 1991;156(1):33–8.
11. Golan A, Tur-Kaspa I. The management of the infertile patient with proximal tubal occlusion. Hum Reprod. 1996;11(9):1833–4.
12. Kosseim M, Brunham RC. Fallopian tube obstruction as a sequela to Chlamydia trachomatis infection. Eur J Clin Microbiol. 1986;5(5):584–90.
13. Saracoglu F, Mungan T, Tanzer F. Salpingitis isthmica nodosa in infertility and ectopic pregnancy. Gynecol Obstet Invest. 1992;34:202–5.
14. Thurmond AS, Brandt KR, Gorrill MJ. Tubal obstruction after ligation reversal surgery: results of catheter recanalization. Radiology. 1999;210(3):747–50.
15. Jenkins CS, Williams SR, Schmidt GE. Salpingitis isthmica nodosa: a review of the literature, discussion of clinical significance, and consideration of patient management. Fertil Steril. 1993;60(4):599–607.
16. Wollcott R. Proximal tubal occlusion: a practical approach. Hum Reprod. 1996;11(9): 1831–3.
17. Evaluating Infertility. American College of Obstetricians and Gynecologists. Washington, DC. November 2007. http://www.acog.org/publications/patient_education/bp136.cfm. Accessed July 15, 2010.
18. Infertility. American Society of Reproductive Medicine. Birmingham, AL, January 2007. http://www.asrm.org. Accessed July 15, 2010.
19. Katz V. Chapter 3: Reproductive anatomy – clinical correlations. In: Katz V, Lobo R, Lentz G, Gershenson D, editors. Comprehensive gynecology. 5th ed. Philadelphia: Mosby; 2007. p. 43–72.
20. Gray H. The female genital organs. In: Gray H, revised by Lewis W, editors. Anatomy of the human body. 20th ed. Philadelphia: Lea & Febiger; 1918; Bartleby.com 2000. http://www. bartleby.com/107/265.html. Accessed August 8, 2010.
21. Kodaman PH, Arici A, Seli E. Evidence-based diagnosis and management of tubal factor infertility. Curr Opin Obstet Gynecol. 2004;16(3):221–9.
22. National Collaborating Centre for Women's and Children's Health. Fertility: assessment and treatment for people with fertility problems. London: RCOG Press; 2004.
23. The Practice Committee for the American Society of Reproductive Medicine. Optimal evaluation of the infertile female. Fertil Steril. 2006;86(5 Suppl 1):S264–7.
24. Brant W. Genital tract: radiographic imaging and MR. In: Brant W, Helms C, editors. Fundamentals of diagnostic radiology. 3rd ed. Philadelphia: Lippincott, Williams & Wilkins; 2007. p. 909–24.
25. ACOG. Practice bulletin no. 104: antibiotic prophylaxis for gynecologic procedures. Obstet Gynecol. 2009;113(5):1180–9.
26. Pinto AB, Hovsepian DM, Wattanakumtornkul S, Pilgram TK. Pregnancy outcomes after fallopian tube recanalization: oil-based versus water-soluble contrast agents. J Vasc Interv Radiol. 2003;14(1):69–74.

27. Silberzweig JE. Incidence of pain during hysterosalpingography using a balloon catheter. AJR Am J Roentgenol. 2007;189:W48.
28. Thurmond AS, Novy M, Uchida BT, Rösch J. Fallopian tube obstruction: selective salpingography and recanalization. Work in progress. Radiology. 1987;163(2):511–4.
29. Thurmond AS, Rosch J. Nonsurgical fallopian tube recanalization for treatment of infertility. Radiology. 1990;174:371–4.
30. Lang EK, Dunaway HH. Recanalization of obstructed fallopian tube by selective salpingography and transvaginal bougie dilatation: outcome and cost analysis. Fertil Steril. 1996;66(2):210–5.
31. Kumpe DA, Zwerdlinger SC, Rothbarth LJ, Durham JD, Albrecht BH. Proximal fallopian tube occlusion: diagnosis and treatment with transcervical fallopian tube catheterization. Radiology. 1990;177(1):183–7.
32. Li QY, Zhou XL, Qin HP, Liu R. [Analysis of 1006 cases with selective salpingography and fallopian tube recanalization]. Zhonghua Fu Chan Ke Za Zhi. 2004;39(2):80–2.
33. Hovsepian DM, Bonn J, Eschelman DJ, Shapiro MJ, Sullivan KL, Gardiner Jr GA. Fallopian tube recanalization in an unrestricted patient population. Radiology. 1994;190(1):137–40.
34. Papaioannou S, Afnan M, Sharif K. The role of selective salpingography and tubal catheterization in the management of the infertile couple. Curr Opin Obstet Gynecol. 2004;16(4):325–9.
35. Papaioannou S, Afnan M, Girling AJ, et al. The effect on pregnancy rates of tubal perfusion pressure reductions achieved by guide-wire tubal catheterization. Hum Reprod. 2002;17(8):2174–9.
36. Thurmond AS. Pregnancies after selective salpingography and tubal recanalization. Radiology. 1994;190(1):11–3.

Fallopian Tube Occlusion

Elizabeth Ann Ignacio, Nadia J. Khati, John C. Lipman,
and Prasanna Vasudevan

Introduction

Presently, there are a multitude of options available to women to control their fertility, depending on changing needs over a lifetime, as well as their health and specific medical conditions. Temporary choices include barrier methods, e.g., the female and male condoms, oral contraceptives, and intrauterine devices. Permanent solutions include sterilization surgery for men or women and, more recently, noninvasive fallopian tube occlusion for women. The efficacy, risks, side effect profile, and cost for each form of contraception are important considerations for each woman. There are many choices for women to consider for contraception. In the United States alone, greater than 11 million women have chosen tubal sterilization as their contraceptive method of choice, with greater than 300,000 women choosing transcervical fallopian tube occlusion [7]. While LTL is the gold standard, more patients will continue to opt for noninvasive techniques such as transcervical fallopian tube occlusion as a simple, safe, and effective solution.

The most widely used form of contraception in the United States is the oral contraceptive pill (OCP). OCPs come in two forms, an estrogen and progestin combination or progestin only formulation. They target the female hormonal cycle to inhibit ovulation. They are a cost-effective way to control fertility; however, their efficacy is strongly dependent on patient compliance. For those seeking long-term contraception, this can be laborious, and missed pills lead to unnecessary worry. The failure rates for OCPs are broken down into expected and typical for this reason. Typical expected failure rates range from 0.1 for combination pills and 0.5–1.25 for progestin-only formulations [1]. OCPs can cause inconvenient side effects such as weight gain, changes in menstrual flow, mood changes, and breast tenderness as well as more serious even dangerous side effects including pulmonary embolus, heart attack, stroke, clotting disorders, and increased risk of cervical and breast cancer. OCPs are inexpensive; however, they represent a monthly cost that will add up over time. While OCPs are a convenient and inexpensive option for some, they are not ideal for long-term or permanent contraception.

Outside of the United States, the intrauterine device (IUD) is the most commonly used form of contraception. The IUD offers semipermanent contraception. There are currently

E.A. Ignacio (✉)
Department of Radiology, Division of Interventional Radiology,
The George Washington University Medical Center, Washington, DC, USA
e-mail: eaignaciomd@gmail.com

E.A. Ignacio and A.C. Venbrux (eds.), *Women's Health in Interventional Radiology*,
DOI 10.1007/978-1-4419-5876-1_4, © Springer Science+Business Media, LLC 2012

two types that are FDA approved in the United States, a copper wire system (Paragard®, Duramed Pharmaceuticals Inc, Pomona, NY) and an IUD whose main mechanism of action is through local levonorgestrel deposition (Mirena®, Bayer HealthCare Pharmaceuticals, Wayne, NJ). IUDs are usually placed in the gynecologist's office during menses but may also be placed postabortion or postpartum; however, the latter comes with an increased risk of uterine perforation. Typically, an IUD can stay in place for up to 5 years, and maintenance consists of a "string check" to ensure that the device was not inadvertently expelled from the uterine cavity. The rate of unintended pregnancy within the first year of typical use in Paragard® patients is 0.8, and in Mirena® patients it is 0.1 [2]. The side effects of Paragard® include bleeding and cramping, whereas Mirena® causes amenorrhea and hormonal complaints. With either form, there is an increased risk of PID in the first 20 days after insertion, with subsequent resultant risk of infertility and ectopic pregnancy [2]. IUDs are highly subsidized, as they are marketed as a viable option in third world countries, and thus are also an affordable option. The IUD offers a more long-term, less expensive option for contraception but comes with its own set of risks. Although it can be placed long term, the IUD is removable, and therefore it is not truly a permanent answer for women.

For those patients who desire an irreversible form of contraception, the current gold standard is laparoscopic tubal ligation (LTL). This technique involves obtaining intra-abdominal access and is usually performed under general anesthesia. Once access is obtained and the fallopian tubes visualized, occlusion is achieved via a variety of surgical methods including electrocoagulation, or multiple different types of bands and/or clips. The intraoperative risks are mostly associated with general anesthesia; however, there is a low risk of damage to major blood vessels, bowel, or the bladder. After the procedure, the patients may experience significant discomfort from the CO_2 used to insufflate the peritoneal cavity during the procedure. There is usually a 48–72 h recovery period where patients experience incisional pain, pain from CO_2 in the peritoneal cavity, and pain from fallopian tube tissue necrosis. Postoperative pain is increased in patients who have received the band or clip method. After the perioperative period, patients generally do not experience discomfort. The failure rate within the first year is about 0.5% [3]. The cost of LTL has been reported between $2880 and $3449 and is a one-time cost [3]. LTL offers a practical but more expensive option for permanent contraception and involves abdominal surgery with significant associated risks.

Since LTL is an invasive procedure, there has been significant research into looking for noninvasive methods to achieve permanent contraception. Focus has been placed on transcervical approaches to ligate or occlude the fallopian tubes.

The first attempts at transcervical sterilization date back to 1878 and were done blind using electrocautery. In 1927, Schroeder postulated using a hysteroscope for direct visualization of the fallopian ostia and documented the first attempts in 1934. At that time, there was a high failure rate and significant intraprocedure risk of uterine perforation and thermal injury to bowel [3].

Another attempted method was thermal occlusion via the neodymium:yttrium-aluminum-garnet laser. While this method did not raise safety concerns as the thermal energy applied only penetrated to a depth of 5 mm, failure rates reached 74%. This method was quickly abandoned once its efficacy became clear [3].

Many different forms of mechanical sterilization have also been explored. Injection of silicone into the tube to form a plug has been used in a small subset of patients. This procedure is expensive, and there is a risk of extravasation of silicone into the paratubal or myometrial tissue. Also, the plug can fracture or the tubes can spasm, requiring a second procedure for placement. For those in whom placement was successful, failure rates are reported as 0.02% [4]. Another form of mechanical contraception, called the P-block device, uses a nylon skeleton with cyanoacrylate to cause both mechanical blockage and fibrosis of the tube. Studies show poor occlusion rates, and there is ongoing research into this device [4].

The only FDA-approved methods of transcervical sterilization in the United States are the Essure® (Conceptus Inc, Mountain View, CA) and Adiana® (Hologic Inc, Bedford, MA) devices.

Designed for hysteroscopic placement, the Interventional Radiologist can place the Essure® device with fluoroscopic guidance off-label. Correct placement and tubal occlusion are confirmed at 12 weeks with hysterosalpingogram. From the hysteroscopic data, successful bilateral placement for Essure® is 98% [5]. The Essure® Micro-insert is 98% effective in preventing pregnancy after 2 years of follow-up. Essure® is more cost effective when compared to LTL, showing an approximate $180 savings per patient for in-office placement versus LTL in an operating room [3].

Adiana® is a form of combined thermal and mechanical occlusion that has been used outside the US and has recently been FDA approved. This hysteroscopic transcervical procedure involves controlled radio-frequency–endocoagulation of the fallopian tube followed by insertion of a silicone matrix within the lumen. Unlike Essure®, Adiana® is not radiopaque and consequently cannot be placed with fluoroscopic guidance. Occlusion is confirmed with a hysterosalpingogram at 3 months as an outpatient. The overall safety of the procedure itself is high. The only complication noted in limited trials was one case of hyponatremia that was treated medically prior to patient discharge. The procedure is well tolerated; 98% of patients tolerated it "well" to "excellent," 25% described "some cramping," and 2% complained of post-procedural pain [3]. There are limited long-term data, as this is a new device. However, 1 year failure rates have been reported as 1.08% and 2 year failure rates as 1.82%, less than that of LTL and Essure®[6].

There are many choices for women to consider for contraception. In the United States alone, greater than 11 million women have chosen tubal sterilization as their contraceptive method of choice, with greater than 300,000 women choosing transcervical fallopian tube occlusion [7]. While LTL is the gold standard, more patients will continue to opt for noninvasive techniques such as transcervical fallopian tube occlusion as a simple, safe, and effective solution.

Anatomy

Female Reproductive Anatomy

Please see the Anatomy section in Chap. 3.

Imaging

Patients do not require any preprocedure imaging for this elective procedure. However, a prospective evaluation of the patient's specific anatomic morphology on imaging does impact the choice for fallopian tube occlusion. For example, hydrosalpinx is not an absolute contraindication, but patients with such documented findings should be informed that the dilated tube may not be favorable anatomy for secure placement of the Essure® device.

Patient Encounter

Indications and Contraindications

Presently, the placement of the Essure® device for fallopian tube occlusion under fluoroscopy by the Interventional Radiologist is off-label, while the Adiana® device is currently only placed via hysteroscopic guidance. This discussion will focus on the Essure® device and the preparation of patients for the Interventional Radiology procedure under fluoroscopic guidance.

The singular indication for fallopian tube occlusion is the desire to end fertility.

Fallopian tube occlusion for sterilization is contraindicated in any patient who is not certain about her desire to end fertility, or who has a proximal tube occlusion or uterine anomaly, e.g., unicornuate uterus, or who has had a previous tubal ligation. Fallopian tube occlusion is further contraindicated in pregnancy or suspected pregnancy, delivery or termination of a pregnancy less than 6 weeks before occlusion device placement, active pelvic infection, allergy to contrast media, or hypersensitivity to nickel confirmed by skin test.

Consult, Consent, and Preparation

A consult visit with the patient is always helpful to discuss the benefits and risks of the device and the procedure.

There are several benefits of fallopian tube occlusion versus other types of permanent sterilization for women. The procedure can be performed safely as an outpatient procedure, and it does not require incisions or general anesthesia. Rates of Essure® technical success, efficacy, and reliability are favorable with a pregnancy prevention rate of greater than 99% [8]. (See Outcomes section in this chapter) Certainly, no method of contraception is 100%. But the Essure® device does have an efficacy rate comparable to that of female surgical tubal ligation.

A discussion of the off-label placement of Essure® via fluoroscopic guidance is essential to full disclosure, although patients should understand that many Interventional Radiology tools are also off-label but still the standard of care. In Interventional Radiology, there are intuitively many real technical advantages of fluoroscopic placement for patients. Smaller delivery devices are used in Interventional Radiology along the order of 5–9 Fr size, particularly compared to the delivery via a 16–20 Fr size hysteroscope. There is also no need for the 1 l of uterine infusate typical of hysteroscopy. With smaller tools and less uterine distension, patient pain and discomfort is likely less. Concomitantly, the sedation or anesthesia requirements with the associated risks may also be substantially reduced. Fluoroscopy does expose the patient to radiation, and this may be concerning for some women. Providing a reasonable prediction of fluoroscopy time and calculated radiation dose is useful for patients to make an informed decision about the procedure.

Patients may expect to experience some of the following clinical symptoms post-procedure with incidences as noted: cramping 30%, pain 13%, nausea/vomiting 11%, dizziness/lightheadedness 9%, bleeding/spotting 7%, vasovagal response/fainting 1.3%, broken device, infection, and anesthesia risks [9]. Overall, the procedure is well tolerated by patients. Most women return to work in 1–2 days.

While there is a high technical success rate, the patient should be warned that the procedure will be terminated if the physician is unable to place an occlusive device in both fallopian tubes. Bilateral placement is important for clinical effectiveness and reliability.

Patients should be instructed regarding the time course for the procedure and the required follow-up imaging study by hysterosalpingogram to confirm fallopian tube occlusion. The waiting period post placement is 3 months, and during that time the patient and partner should rely on an alternative form of birth control.

Patients who have had radio-frequency endometrial ablation and subsequent formation of uterine synechiae may not accurately be assessed with the required 3 month follow-up hysterosalpingogram, and therefore should not be advised to undergo concomitant fallopian tube occlusion with Essure®.

Special consideration should be made for patients with a medical history of the recent use of corticosteroids. Immunosuppressant therapy may inhibit the normal inflammatory response to the occlusion device and tissue ingrowth needed for effective tube occlusion. These patients who are candidates for Essure® placement should be counseled that it may take longer than 3 months to reach device efficacy. An alternative form of birth control is always required until imaging confirmation of tubal occlusion.

Patient Preparation

The patient should schedule her procedure during the first half of her menstrual cycle, thereby decreasing the risk of an undiagnosed pregnancy at the time of the procedure. This may also help with visualization of the fallopian tube on during the procedure.

A negative serum pregnancy test may be acquired on the day of the procedure. Given the use of fluoroscopy, this is a medical–legal requirement at the authors' institution.

Patients are advised to take a nonsteroidal anti-inflammatory medication before the procedure. Ibuprofen 800 mg p.o. 1–2 h before the procedure is a frequent choice. Some physicians recommend ketorolac before or during the procedure. The use of preprocedure NSAIDS provides the dual purpose of analgesia as well as decreased tubal spasm.

Prophylaxis with antibiotics may be achieved with oral doxycycline 100 mg, one tablet by mouth twice a day beginning 2 days before the procedure, the day of the procedure, and for 2 days after the procedure (ten tablets dispensed).

Technique

Equipment and Materials

Vaginal Speculum

Disposable plastic vaginal specula are available in sizes small, medium, and large. A light source is needed, and there are some disposable specula with an attached LED light that are especially helpful for direct visualization of the cervix. A metallic speculum may be used; however, metal is radiopaque and limits visualization of the vaginal vault under fluoroscopy.

Guide Sheath

A transcervical sheath may be used. To accommodate the Essure® delivery catheter, the guide sheath must be at least 5 Fr size. Some authors prefer the 9 Fr (3 mm diameter) Intrauterine Access Balloon catheter (Cook Medical Inc, Bloomington, IN), which is excellent for maintaining access during the procedure. A sidearm is present in order to flush or inject contrast during the entire procedure.

Operators may also choose a directional guiding sheath/catheter such as a 7 Fr renal double curve. Again, a sideport is present to allow for flush or contrast injection.

Essure® Occlusion Device

The occlusive device is the coil or Micro-insert with two components: there is a stainless steel inner core with polyester fibers and a nitinol outer anchoring core. The Micro-insert measures 3.5 cm long and expands to a diameter of 2 mm when released. Four radiopaque markers are present in order to position the device properly with fluoroscopic guidance (Fig. 4.1).

Presently, the Essure® device manufactured by Conceptus is the only FDA-approved device available for fallopian tube occlusion that has radiopaque markers to facilitate fluoroscopic placement. By design, this device was originally made to be deployed under hysteroscopy. For the Interventional Radiologist, the use of fluoroscopy for visualization and deployment is presently off-label.

Catheter

The Essure® disposable delivery catheter is 4.3 Fr and consists of a handle, a delivery wire, release catheter, delivery catheter, and the Essure® Micro-insert (Fig. 4.2).

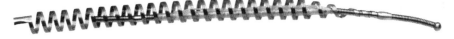

Fig. 4.1 Essure® Micro-insert (Courtesy of Conceptus, Inc. With permission)

Fig. 4.2 Essure® Delivery
Catheter (Courtesy of
Conceptus, Inc. With
permission)

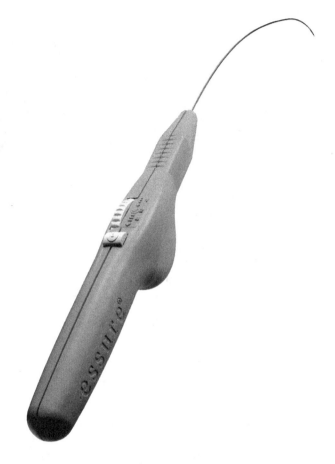

Procedure Start

The technique is relatively straightforward, similar to that of fallopian tube recanalization
and requiring the same skill set. Although designed for delivery under hysteroscopy, the
following discussion will review the fluoroscopic technique of Essure® placement for the
Interventional Radiologist only.

The procedure may be performed in the standard Interventional Radiology suite with
fluoroscopy. Procedure time may be approximately 30 min, depending on the patient's
anatomy. The patient lies supine with the lower extremities in the open lithotomy position, similar to that for a pelvic examination. The patient's knees may be flexed laterally
(frog leg), and/or one may use surgical stirrups for support depending on the patient's
comfort.

Anesthesia may be achieved with intravenous sedation, e.g., midazolam. Paracervical
block is also an option, but not usually necessary. Some operators instruct outpatients to
take an anti-inflammatory (typically 800 mg of ibuprofen p.o. or even ketorolac) 2 h before

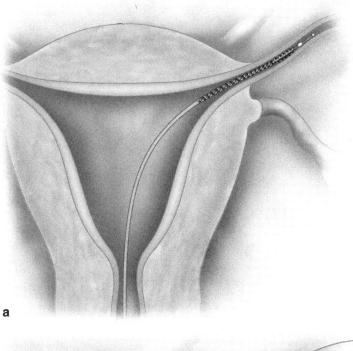

a

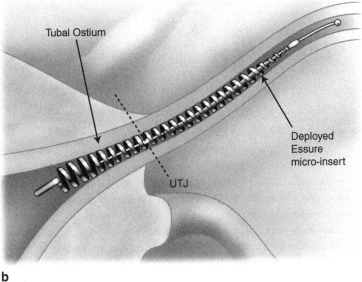

b

Fig. 4.3 (**a, b**) Essure® (Conceptus, Inc., Mountain View, CA) placement

their procedure appointment for analgesia. Once anesthesia and/or sedation are achieved, the perineum may be prepped. The perineum can be prepped with povidone/iodine scrub (Purdue Products, Stamford, CT) or even a baby shampoo/mild detergent. The area is then covered with sterile blue towels and a paper drape in the usual fashion.

Step by Step

A bivalved speculum is inserted into the vagina and locked in place for the procedure. The guide sheath can be placed transcervical using a soft J tip guide wire.

The procedure begins with a hysterosalpingogram. The technique for the initial hysterosalpingogram has been discussed. (See Chap. 3.) Both fallopian tubes should be identified at the start of the procedure.

A roadmap image of the uterus, fallopian tube ostium, and proximal tubal segment may be obtained by contrast injection from the sidearm of the guide sheath. This imaging will help with precise placement of the delivery catheter.

The Essure® delivery catheter is placed at the selected fallopian tube, and the device is advanced until the third marker is at the tubal ostium (Fig. 4.3a, b). One advances the Essure® delivery system into the proximal fallopian tube with slow, steady forward movement to prevent tubal spasm. For optimal placement, the Essure® Micro-insert should span the intramural and the proximal isthmic segments of the fallopian tube, with the outer coil spanning the uterotubal junction (UTJ). To achieve ideal positioning, one may retract the delivery catheter and the release catheter using the thumbwheel on the handle (Fig. 4.4). The button allows the physician to change the function of the thumbwheel from retracting the delivery catheter to retracting the release catheter. The delivery wire is detached from the Micro-insert by rotating the system [10].

With the device handle in a stable position, one rotates the thumbwheel on the handle toward the operator, no faster than 1 click per second until the wheel no longer rotates. This facilitates withdrawal of the delivery catheter and exposes the wound-down Essure® Micro-insert attached to the release catheter. Approximately 1 cm of the Micro-insert should appear trailing into the uterus when the delivery catheter is withdrawn.

Once the delivery catheter is retracted, one depresses the button on the handle to enable the thumbwheel to be further rotated. With rotation, the release catheter is withdrawn. This allows the outer coil of the Micro-insert to expand. In some instances, the Micro-insert can jump forward about 1 mm, so one should make allowance for this possibility. For optimal placement, it is best to place the third radiopaque landmark at the tubal ostium [11].

The operator should wait approximately 10 s to allow the outer coils to fully expand. Once the outer coils are expanded, one turns the entire handle counterclockwise at least 10 rotations while gently pulling backward on the handle to release the delivery wire from the Micro-insert. The delivery system can now be fully removed from the patient (Fig. 4.5).

Occasionally, resistance is met, which may indicate that the device is not concentrically aligned in the fallopian tube. If gentle pressure does not allow for advancement of the device, then the procedure should be terminated to avoid either uterine perforation or

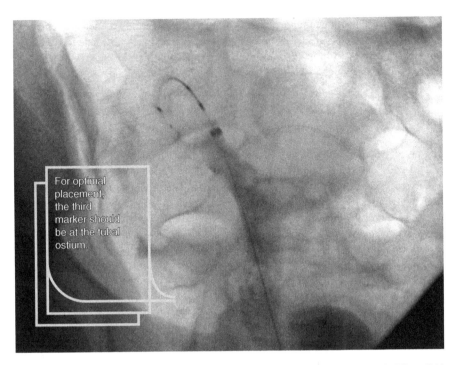

For optimal placement, the third marker should be at the tubal ostium.

Fig. 4.4 Transcervical sheath. Essure® delivery catheter (Conceptus, Inc., Mountain View, CA) advanced into right fallopian tube. One may retract using the thumbwheel for ideal positioning of the third radiopaque marker

inadvertent deployment of the Micro-insert into the uterine musculature rather than the tubal lumen. If the angle to the fallopian tube is not favorable for centrally positioning the Essure® catheter at the ostium, the coaxial use of a directional catheter such as a 6 Fr renal double curve catheter may facilitate placement.

One Micro-insert is placed in each fallopian tube. Manufacturer recommendations state that if bilateral microcoils cannot be placed, then the procedure should be aborted.

Once each Micro-insert is in place, some operators will take final contrast injection images as well as non-contrast images in order to confirm placement and document position for comparison with post images that will be done 3 months later.

All catheters, wires, sheath, and speculum are removed at the end of the procedure.

Hints, Technical Pitfalls, and Pearls

If the Micro-insert is too far distal, the manufacturer does not recommend overlapping the device. Further, the manufacturer warns that removal should not be attempted once the Micro-insert has been placed, unless >80% of the length (18 or more coils) of the Essure® Micro-insert is trailing into the uterine cavity, as this may result in fallopian tube perforation or other patient injury.

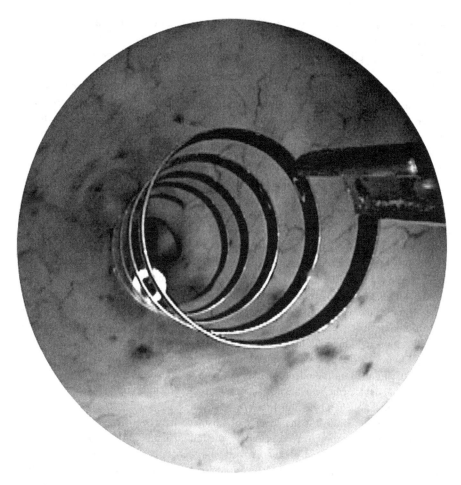

Fig. 4.5 Hysteroscopic image immediately post placement; Micro-insert (Essure®) in place (Courtesy of Conceptus, Inc. With permission)

Certainly, if the Micro-insert was inadvertently deployed in the uterine cavity and not into the tube, then the Micro-insert can be removed from the uterus and another attempt made at Micro-insert placement in the tube. The Micro-insert that is free in the uterine cavity may be captured with a gooseneck snare system placed through the guide sheath.

Postoperative Care, Discharge Instructions, and Follow-Up

Post procedure and depending on sedation, a patient can be discharged home 1 h after the procedure is completed. Discharge instructions must include a scheduled follow-up hysterosalpingogram (HSG) in 3 months in order to confirm complete occlusion of each tube. During the 3 month waiting period after the procedure, couples are counseled to use another form of birth control. The 3-month follow-up HSG is a strict requirement [10]. Patient compliance with follow-up imaging is important for established device efficacy.

The outer and inner coils of the Essure® device have characteristic radiodense markers that are easily visualized at radiography and fluoroscopy. The two most proximal markers (at the uterine cornua) correspond to the proximal outer coil and proximal inner coil, respectively. The two most distal markers (in the distal fallopian tube) correspond to the distal end of the outer and inner coils, respectively (Fig. 4.1). According to the device manufacturers, the HSG protocol post-Essure® placement includes injection of radiodense contrast material into the uterine cavity using a low-flow and low-pressure method in order to minimize patient discomfort (cramping and possible vasovagal reaction) and also to avoid dislodging the device from its position if the contrast is injected too fast [10].

The device manufacturers recommend obtaining a minimum of six radiographs at the time of the procedure: a scout radiograph; early minimal fill of the uterus; partial fill of the uterus; complete fill of the uterine cavity; and bilateral magnification views of the uterine cornua. All images of the uterine cavity should ideally be captured in the anteroposterior rather than the fundal projection so as to visualize the bilateral cornua [10]. As noted previously, the contrast is injected through the catheter using a low-flow and low-pressure technique. Position and function of the device can then be assessed.

The Essure® device is properly placed when the Micro-insert crosses the uterotubal junction. Using the four radiodense markers of both inner and outer coils, adequate positioning of the device can be evaluated according to their relationship to the cornua of the uterus and the fallopian tubes (Fig. 4.6a–f).

Assessing the position of the inner coil (distance between the second and fourth radiodense markers from the uterine cavity to the fallopian tube) is most important since it hosts the PET fibers which induce fibrosis and, hence, occlusion. According to the Essure® physician training manual [10], a grade of 1, 2, and 3 is used to categorize the device's position: expulsion into the uterine cavity or too proximal (grade 1); satisfactory position (grade 2); and too distal position or expelled into the peritoneal cavity (grade 3). Adequate position (grade 2) is achieved when the Micro-insert crosses the uterotubal junction, with the proximal end of the inner coil (second marker from the uterine cavity to the tubes) visualized within 30 mm from the filled uterine cornua or when less than half of the length of the inner coil is seen trailing into the uterine cavity. The distal ends of the outer and inner coils (third and fourth radiodense markers, respectively, from the uterine cavity to the tubes) should be seen within the distal aspects of the fallopian tubes (Fig. 4.7). After placement of the device, the coils can migrate proximally and be expulsed into the uterine cavity (grade 1), or distally along the tube and be expelled into the peritoneal cavity (grade 3). Both of these grades are considered unsatisfactory. At HSG, grade 1 is defined as either non-visualization of the device (presumably due to expulsion through the uterine cavity) or as more than half of the inner coil (distance between the second and fourth radiodense markers) seen trailing into the uterine cavity (Fig. 4.8). Grade 3 is when the device no longer crosses the uterotubal junction with the proximal end of the inner coil (second radiodense marker) more than 30 mm

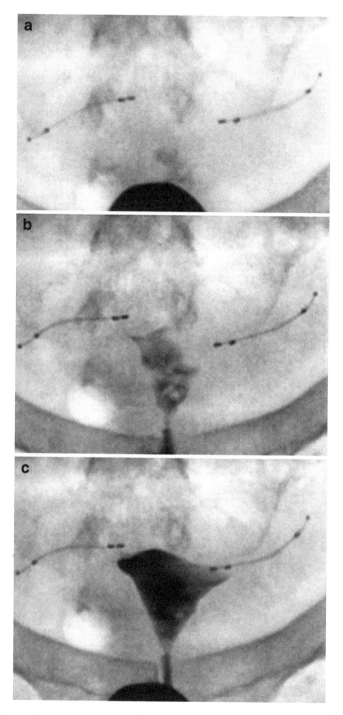

Fig. 4.6 (a–f) Follow-up hysterosalpingogram after 3 months. Bilateral Essure® Micro-inserts (Conceptus, Inc., Mountain View, CA) in good position. (**a**) Scout. (**b**) Minimal filling. (**c**) Partial filling. (**d**) Complete filling. (**e**) Magnified view of left cornua. (**f**) Magnified view of right cornua (Courtesy of Conceptus, Inc. With permission)

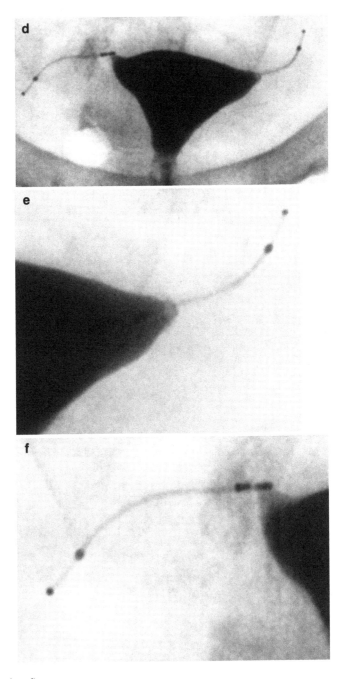

Fig. 4.6 (continued)

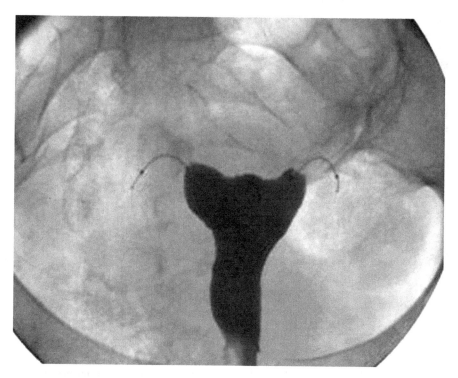

Fig. 4.7 Fallopian tube occlusion

distal in the tube from the distended contrast-filled uterine cornua (Fig. 4.9) or if the device is seen within the peritoneal cavity.

In addition to confirming position of the device, the 3-month follow-up HSG evaluates its function by demonstrating tubal occlusion. Since the inner portion of the coil is the one hosting the PET fibers that induce the chronic fibrosis responsible for tubal occlusion, one can infer that any degree of inner coil malposition could result in malfunction of the device. Similarly to device's position, tubal occlusion may be graded on a scale of 1–3 according to Essure® physician training manual [10]. Grade 1 is defined as occlusion of the tube at the uterine cornua; grade 2 is defined when there is opacification of the tube but no extension of the contrast beyond the distal portion of the outer coil (third radiodense marker on radiographs), and grade 3 is defined as opacification of the tube past the Micro-insert with or without free intraperitoneal spillage.

Correct interpretation of the HSG by radiologists is paramount because patients are managed differently depending on the device's position and proper function. When the Essure® device is correctly located at the uterotubal junction (grade 2) and both tubes are occluded (grades 1 or 2), the patient can rely on it as the sole means of contraception. If it crosses the uterotubal junction (grade 2) but tubal occlusion is not achieved (grade 3),

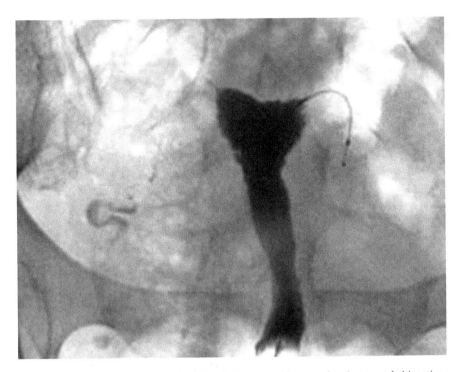

Fig. 4.8 Only the left device is visualized in satisfactory position crossing the uterotubal junction. Left tubal occlusion was satisfactory. The right Micro-insert (Essure®, Conceptus, Inc., Mountain View, CA) was not identified on the scout HSG radiograph, presumed to have been expulsed into the uterine cavity. There is contrast opacification of the right fallopian tube

patients are scheduled for another 3-month follow-up HSG to allow additional time for the fibrosis to develop around the coil. During that time, patients should continue using alternative means of contraception. Any combination of device's abnormal position (grades 1 or 3) with or without tubal occlusion alters the management of each patient. They should be instructed not to rely on the device and to continue using alternative means of contraception, consider repositioning of the Micro-inserts, or opt for surgical sterilization. The presence or absence of tubal blockage does not modify management in cases of device abnormal position.

This grading system is helpful as it combines a description of the device's location as well as its function, thereby providing clinicians and their patients with an easy and quick management algorithm. Further education of radiologists performing the 3-month follow-up HSG is needed in order to be more familiar with the appearance of the device on radiographs, be able to recognize each of the radiodense markers of the coils, and appreciate the presence of small wisps of contrast that may extend beyond the distal end of the device.

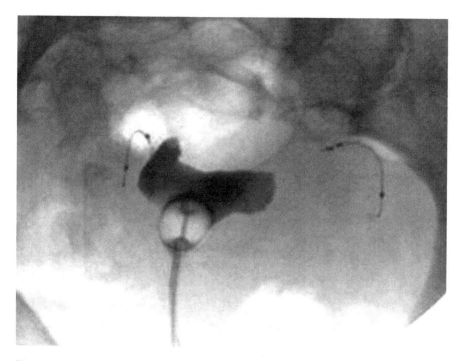

Fig. 4.9 The left Micro-insert (Essure®, Conceptus, Inc., Mountain View, CA) coil is too distal in location. The proximal portion does not cross the uterotubal junction. Despite the abnormal position, there was no opacification of the left tube. The right Micro-insert is also slightly too distal

Alternative Imaging for Confirmation

As the Essure® device is becoming a more prevalent form of permanent female birth control, it will be more commonly encountered in patients who are undergoing other imaging examinations for various reasons. Radiologists should be able to recognize the device on other cross-sectional imaging studies such as computed tomography (CT) and magnetic resonance imaging (MRI) scans. The device has a characteristic appearance on both CT scans (Fig. 4.10a, b) and MRI (Fig. 4.11a, b). It should be noted that neither of these two imaging modalities are currently used to assess for the device's position or function.

In Europe and Australia, investigators advocate using a single pelvic radiograph or transvaginal pelvic ultrasound (US) to replace the 3-month follow-up HSG in the evaluation of proper device position [12–14]. The potential benefits of using either of these two imaging modalities over HSG include decreased or no radiation to the patient; avoiding the use of a contrast agent and its related possible reaction; less patient discomfort; and

Fig. 4.10 (a, b) Axial CT scan pelvis with soft tissue windows (a) And bone windows (b). The right Micro-insert (Essure®, Conceptus, Inc., Mountain View, CA) is easily visualized as a linear hyperdense structure extending from the uterine cornua to the proximal fallopian tube. The radiodense markers are better identified on the bone window settings

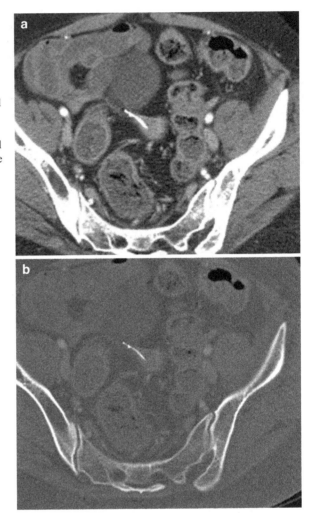

better patient compliance. The main problem with these two modalities is that neither of them can assess for tubal occlusion. In addition, pelvic radiography can document the absence or presence and relative symmetry of the Essure® device in the pelvis with the limitation of providing its relationship to the uterine cornua and fallopian tubes. Nevertheless, replacing the 3-month follow-up HSG confirmation test with a pelvic US seems very attractive to patients and their physician as shown by prior investigators [12, 14] due to its lack of ionizing radiation, its ease of reproducibility, its cost-effectiveness, and because it ensures better patient compliance. The added use of 3D pelvic ultrasound to the conventional two-dimensional US may allow for better visualization of the device in its entirety in the reconstructed coronal plane. The coils are visualized on US (Fig. 4.12) and appear as echogenic linear structures distinguished from surrounding soft tissue structures, which should extend from the uterine cornua to the proximal tubes.

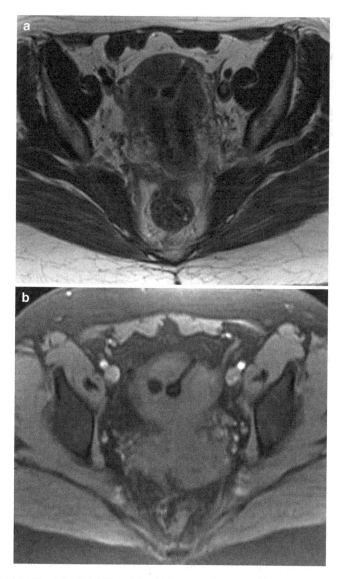

Fig. 4.11 (**a, b**) MRI pelvis. Axial T2 weighted (**a**) And axial T1 weighted (**b**) Fat-saturated image through the pelvis. Both right and left Micro-inserts (Essure®, Conceptus, Inc., Mountain View, CA) are seen as signal void crossing the uterotubal junction

Legendre et al. have developed a classification system [15] describing the relationship of the coils to the cornua and tubes. They correlated their findings of coil location on US with findings of location and tubal occlusion at HSG. They found that only coils that had migrated distally in the tube and were no longer crossing the uterotubal junction showed evidence of tubal patency at HSG, concluding that only those patients with very distal coils should undergo HSG and should be managed subsequently depending on the results.

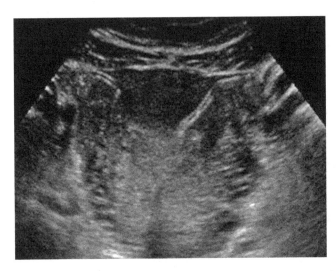

Fig. 4.12 Axial transabdominal sonographic image of the pelvis through the uterine fundus. Both right and left Micro-inserts (Essure®, Conceptus, Inc., Mountain View, CA) are visualized as parallel echogenic lines which have a spring coil appearance corresponding to the outer coil of the device. The inner coil is also usually identified although better seen on real-time studies due to its smaller size

These results seem promising for Essure® patients as they might increase compliance of the device and perhaps decrease the rate of unwanted pregnancies.

Hysterosalpingogram remains the gold standard for evaluation of Essure® fallopian tube occlusion and is most reliable for verifying the effectiveness of this device.

Outcomes

The use of transcervical tubal occlusion for sterilization has become increasingly more popular given the ease of placement and brief recovery period. To date, more than 300,000 women have had fallopian tube occlusion procedures in the United States. As expected, there is a large amount of gynecologic literature covering the hysteroscopic placement of the Essure® and Adiana® devices. However, Interventional Radiology data regarding the fallopian tube occlusion technique under fluoroscopic guidance are limited. Given the paucity of data with regard to fluoroscopic placement, technical success, and complications, no definitive conclusion can yet be drawn and more patient studies are certainly needed.

Similarly, the clinical data regarding safety, efficacy, and patient satisfaction with transcervical methods of tubal occlusion are derived primarily from the data on device placement under hysteroscopy. Review of this literature may still be helpful for the Interventional Radiologist, as the patients' outcomes once fallopian occlusion has been documented are ostensibly the same.

With regard to technical success under fluoroscopic guidance, McSwain et al. reported a success rate of 87.5% in a small series of eight patients [11]. Although the patient number is quite low, these results are concordant to the Phase III clinical trials by Conceptus in 2003, which included 518 sexually active reproductive-age women. Here, Cooper et al. reported that hysteroscopic technical success of bilateral placement rate was 86% on first attempt and 90% on second attempt [16]. A similar success rate of 88.4% has been reported for the Adiana device as well [8, 17].

McSwain et al. postulated that there may be some advantages to fluoroscopic placement over hysteroscopy. They discussed the sequential use of 0.018 and 0.035 in. angle-tipped glide wires in three patients in whom the Essure® device would not primarily pass for placement. With coaxial wire manipulation under fluoroscopic guidance, the Essure® device tracked in the fallopian tubes without difficulty and successfully deployed [11].

Complications

McSwain et al. also reported an immediate complication rate of 12.5% corresponding to one patient who had post-procedure pelvic pain not relieved by nonsteroidal anti-inflammatory medications. Follow-up imaging on this patient had demonstrated accurate placement of the Micro-insert, and post-op pain was attributed to use of a cervical tenaculum [11]. Adverse clinical events reported by Cooper et al. post Essure® with hysteroscopy included four perforations of the uterine wall (1.1%), 14 expulsions (2.9%), and three patients with proximal implant location (0.6%) [16].

After placement using hysteroscopy, most patients may expect to experience cramping (29.6%) and abdominal pain (12.9%). Other symptoms such as nausea/vomiting (10.8%), dizziness/lightheadedness (8.8%), and bleeding/spotting (6.8%) occur to a lesser extent [10]. To date, the experience with the Adiana® system is extremely limited, with only 12 month data. However, as with the Essure® implants, the Adiana® system appears to be well tolerated with low post-procedure clinical events [17].

The Essure® Micro-insert is 98% effective in preventing pregnancy after 2 years follow-up. For Adiana®, the 1 year pregnancy prevention rate as derived with life-table methods was 98.9%. By comparison, the rate of pregnancy with male sterilization surgery is 0.15%, and for female sterilization surgery it is 0.5% [18].

Summary and Conclusions

Today, several options exist for women who desire contraception. Some women specifically seek permanent sterilization, and alternative methods exist and are growing. As a noninvasive procedure, fallopian tube occlusion under fluoroscopic guidance is an attractive choice. For operators, the catheter manipulations are straightforward and may be accomplished with a high level of success. For patients, both the Essure® and Adiana®

devices appear to be equally effective in the prevention of pregnancy. More patient data are needed to compare complication rates post-fluoroscopic placement of these devices, as well as to assess the specific efficacy of subsequent occlusion in achieving permanent sterilization. However, there may be some special advantages in fluoroscopic-guided fallopian occlusion, particularly in those patients who fail placement by conventional hysteroscopic techniques.

References

1. Frye CA. An overview of oral contraceptives: mechanism of action and clinical use. Neurology. 2006;66:S29–36.
2. Macisaac L, Espey E. Intrauterine contraception: the pendulum swings back. Obstet Gynecol Clin North Am. 2007;34(1):91–111.
3. Greenberg JA. Hysteroscopic sterilization: history and current methods. Rev Obstet Gynecol. 2009;1(3):113–21.
4. Abbott J. Transcervical sterilization. Curr Opin Obstet Gynecol. 2007;19:325–30.
5. Connor VF. Essure: a review six years later. J Minim Invasive Gynecol. 2009;16(3):282–90.
6. Smith RD. Contemporary hysteroscopic methods for female sterilization. Int J Gynecol Obstet. 2010;108:79–84.
7. Theroux R. The hysteroscopic approach to sterilization. J Obstet Gynecol Neonatal Nurs. 2008;37:356–60.
8. Palmer SN, Greenberg JA. Transcervical sterilization: a comparison of Essure permanent birth control system and Adiana permanent contraception system. Rev Obstet Gynecol. 2009;2(2):84–92.
9. Kerin JF, Cooper JM, Price T, et al. Hysteroscopic sterilization using a micro-insert device: results of a multicentre Phase II study. Hum Reprod. 2003;18:1223–30.
10. Essure physician training manual: HSG protocol. San Carlos, CA Conceptus, 2002.
11. McSwain H, Shaw C, Hall LD. Placement of the Essure permanent birth control device with fluoroscopic guidance: a novel method for tubal sterilization. J Vasc Interv Radiol. 2005; 16(7):1007–12.
12. Weston G, Bowditch J. Office ultrasound should be the first-line investigation for confirmation of correct ESSURE placement. Aust N Z J Obstet Gynaecol. 2005;45(4):312–5.
13. Teoh M, Meagher S, Kovacs G. Ultrasound detection of the Essure permanent birth control device: a case series. Aust N Z J Obstet Gynaecol. 2003;43(5):378–80.
14. Veersema S, Vleugels MP, Timmermans A, Brölmann HA. Follow-up of successful bilateral placement of Essure microinserts with ultrasound. Fertil Steril. 2005;84(6):1733–6.
15. Legendre G, Gervaise A, Levaillant JM, et al. Assessment of three-dimensional ultrasound examination classification to check the position of the tubal sterilization microinsert. Fertil Steril. 2010;94:2732–5.
16. Cooper JM, Carignan CS, Cher D, Kerin JF. Microinsert nonincisional hysteroscopic sterilization. Obstet Gynecol. 2003;102:59–67.
17. Vancaillie TG, Anderson TL, Johns DA. A 12-month prospective evaluation of transcervical sterilization using implantable polymer matrices. Obstet Gynecol. 2008;112(6):1270–7.
18. U.S. Food and Drug Administration, Centers for Devices and Radiological Health, Guidance for Industry - Uniform Contraceptive Labeling, July 23, 1998, http://www.fda.gov/cdrh/ode/contrlab.html, accessed on 09/05/2011.

Part III

Spine Interventions

Kyphoplasty and Vertebroplasty

5

Jozef M. Brozyna, Denis Primakov, Anthony C. Venbrux,
Ajay D. Wadgaonkar, Sarah LaFond, Jay Karajgikar, and Wayne J. Olan

Introduction

Interventional Radiology has played an increasingly critical role in the arena of women's health. Specifically in the spine, image-guided interventions consist primarily of vertebroplasty, kyphoplasty, spine biopsy, and pain management. The evolution of vertebroplasty and kyphoplasty have changed the management of osteoporotic and malignant vertebral body compression fractures (VCFs), This chapter will discuss each intervention, with particular emphasis given to step-by-step descriptions of the procedures.

Pathophysiology

An estimated 700,000 vertebral collapses occur each year in the United States. Most of these fractures occur in postmenopausal women secondary to osteoporosis. In fact, women over the age of 50 have a 26% chance of having a vertebral compression fracture. This incidence increases with age, climbing to 40% in women over the age of 80. Women who have sustained a previous vertebral fracture have a 19.2% chance of developing new fractures in the following year [1].

The majority of vertebral insufficiency across both genders stems from osteoporosis. Consequently, approximately 70% (68.9%) of back pain associated with vertebral compression fractures is due to osteoporosis. Other less common causes of vertebral compression fractures include metastatic cancer (20.4% of fractures), trauma (4.8%), plasmacytoma or multiple myeloma (4.5%), and symptomatic angioma (1.4%) [2]. See Fig. 5.1.

While completely accurate statistics are not available, it is believed that at least one half of all individuals who die from cancer each year have skeletal metastases. The medical, economic, and social consequences of breast cancer metastasis to the spine can be more severe than any other cause of VCF. In women, breast cancer is the most likely malignancy to metastasize to bone [3, 4]. Just like any other vertebral fracture, a spine metastasis

A.C. Venbrux (✉)
Department of Radiology, Division of Interventional Radiology,
The George Washington University Medical Center, Washington, DC, USA
e-mail: avenbrux@mfa.gwu.edu

E.A. Ignacio and A.C. Venbrux (eds.), *Women's Health in Interventional Radiology*,
DOI 10.1007/978-1-4419-5876-1_5, © Springer Science+Business Media, LLC 2012

Fig. 5.1 Lateral lumbar spine radiograph.
Compression fracture. There is osteopenia and loss
of height in the L2 vertebral body

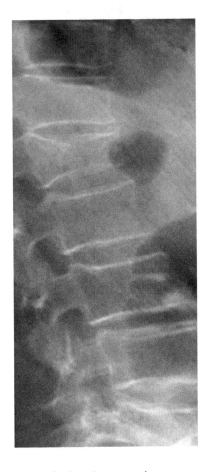

fracture has the potential to induce great pain and cause spinal cord compression, among
other problems. However, metastasized breast cancer cells create a higher propensity for
vertebral compression fracture by promoting osteoclast formation, resulting in increased
bone resorption. In turn, this increased bone resorption can lead to severe and potentially
fatal hypercalcemia.

It is important to note that while spine metastases due to breast cancer are usually osteolytic lesions, osteoblastic activity can also be present and is predominant in 15–20% of
bone metastasis cases [5, 6]. In cases of multiple myeloma, on the other hand, the lesions
are solely osteolytic.

Anatomy

Anatomy of the Spine

There are 7 cervical (C1–C7), 12 thoracic (T1–T12), 5 lumbar (L1–L5), 5 sacral (S1–S5),
and 3–5 coccygeal vertebrae (Fig. 5.2a–d). The sacral and coccygeal vertebrae are fused,
while the superior 24 are moveable to varying degrees and are separated by intervertebral

disks. The cervical spine and the lumbar spine maintain a slight lordotic curvature, while the thoracic and sacral portions of the spine typically maintain a slight kyphotic angulation. See Fig. 5.2a–d.

The cervical spine is distinguished by two unique vertebrae, the "atlas" (C1) and the "axis" (C2), which support and allow for the extreme mobility of the head. *Cervical vertebrae* are the smallest in size and are the only vertebrae to possess a transverse foramen. *Thoracic vertebrae* are intermediate in size and are distinguished by the presence of costal facets for articulation with the ribs. The five *lumbar vertebrae* are the largest and possess none of the above features. From a practical standpoint, the pedicles of the lumbar vertebral bodies are angulated more posterolaterally than in the thoracic spine and thus require a more oblique positioning in order to be visualized on fluoroscopy. The pedicles of the lumbar vertebral bodies are also the thickest and are thus the least challenging to cannulate. Performing spinal augmentation becomes much more difficult as you move up the spine. Fortuitously, compression fractures in the cervical and upper thoracic spine are much less common than in the lower thoracic and lumbar spine.

Variants, such as the presence of four or six lumbar-type vertebral bodies (formed when the L5 is fused with the sacrum, known as sacralization of L5) and underdevelopment of the 12th ribs, are fairly common. This may lead to confusion during reporting of the imaging studies, where the level of injury may be misrepresented. The authors therefore advocate counting the vertebrae under direct fluoroscopic observation prior to performing any spinal intervention in order to ensure that the procedure is performed at the correct spinal level.

Imaging

Review of available imaging studies assists in procedure planning, triaging patients with specific indications and contraindications to vertebroplasty and kyphoplasty. This includes any radiographs, magnetic resonance imaging (MRI) scans, and computed tomography (CT) scans.

Classic findings suggestive of a VCF on radiographs include loss of vertebral body height at the superior and/or inferior vertebral end plates. There is often a wedge appearance from more narrowing and loss of height anteriorly (Fig. 5.1). Radiographs or plain films can also be taken with the patient in different positions to assess the mobility of the vertebrae. However, the relative age of the fracture cannot be determined from spine radiographs.

Characterization and dating of the fractures becomes increasingly important in the geriatric population as many of these patients present with several vertebral fractures, and differentiating which fracture is responsible for their present symptoms is crucial.

MRI is superior in detailing the vertebral anatomy as well as demonstrating marrow signal changes in order to determine the age of the fracture. Sagittal T2-weighted images and short T1 inversion recovery (STIR) sequences are particularly useful in identifying fluid and edema, and thus distinguishing between acute, subacute, and chronic fractures (Fig. 5.3). Acute and subacute fractures that are less than 1 month old will have hypointense T1 signal and hyperintense T2 signal. As the VCF heals, the marrow signal on T1- and T2-weighted images will usually return to normal. Occasionally, the chronic VCF will be hypointense on both T1- and T2-weighted images, indicating bony fibrosis and/or bony sclerosis. Stallmeyer et al. recommends obtaining a CT scan for confirmation of bony sclerosis, as cement injection here would be nearly impossible [7].

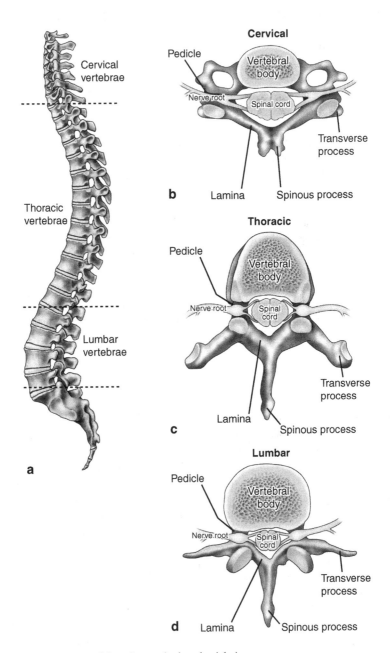

Fig. 5.2 (**a–d**) Anatomy of the spine, sagittal, and axial views

Fig. 5.3 MRI lumbar spine. The patient had acute lower back pain, but several compression fractures, age unknown. Evaluation of STIR sequence reveals the most recent acute fracture at L2. This corresponded to point tenderness on the patient's physical examination (Courtesy of Christopher Neal, MD)

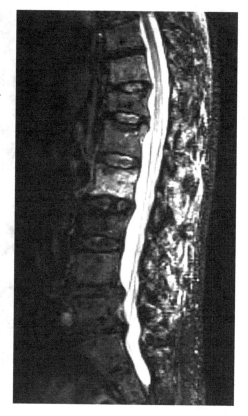

Patients with osteonecrosis of the spine or Kummel Disease may have distinctive MRI features. A fluid collection may be present at the superior end plate, showing T1 hypointense and T2 hyperintense signal. Unlike an infectious process, adjacent inflammatory changes will be absent with Kummel Disease [7].

Thin-section computed tomography (CT) scans are excellent for providing bony detail and will identify the fracture plane throughout the vertebral body, especially if there is extension of the fracture line through the wall. Such a defect may allow extrusion of cement to the spinal canal, and serious caution is advised for spinal interventions in this setting.

Both sagittal and axial MRI or thin-section CT scan can reveal the presence of severe retropulsion of bony fragments. Such a finding is a relative contraindication to vertebroplasty and kyphoplasty as the placement of bone cement might further force the bone fragment(s) posteriorly into the neural canal and result in a "fixed" cord compression. See Fig. 5.4.

If imaging shows evidence of vertebral body end plate destruction adjacent to a disc, disc infection (i.e., discitis) must be investigated. Consideration for vertebroplasty and kyphoplasty should be put on hold. Disc aspiration biopsy is indicated. Culture results will dictate antibiotic therapy and the feasibility of future vertebral body augmentation.

Fig. 5.4 MRI lumbar spine. There are retropulsed fragments present. This is a relative contraindication for spinal augmentation

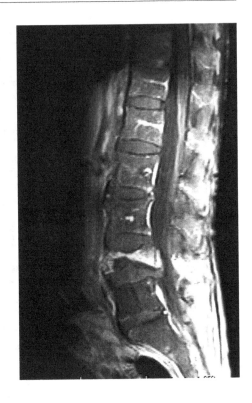

Patient Encounter

Indications and Contraindications

The main indication for vertebroplasty and kyphoplasty is a vertebral body compression fracture (VCF). Studies indicate that between one-third and two-thirds of patients with symptomatic osteoporotic VCFs can achieve back pain relief with conservative medical treatment such as analgesics, bed rest, external fixation, and rehabilitation. The remainder of these patients, the majority of whom are women, continue to suffer from persistent pain and functional restrictions until more invasive treatment is performed [8, 9]. This data, combined with the ever-growing elderly population, make it extremely important for physicians to be knowledgeable about vertebroplasty and kyphoplasty.

As with all image-guided interventions, appropriate patient selection for vertebroplasty and kyphoplasty is essential. In women's health, these techniques are most frequently employed to treat symptomatic osteoporotic vertebral compression fractures in which conservative medical management was attempted for 3–4 weeks and failed. However, osteonecrosis (Kummell Disease) is also an optimal indication for vertebroplasty and kyphoplasty as the cavity can be filled easily with bone cement. Fractures stemming from multiple myeloma and spine metastases can also be treated with either procedure [1].

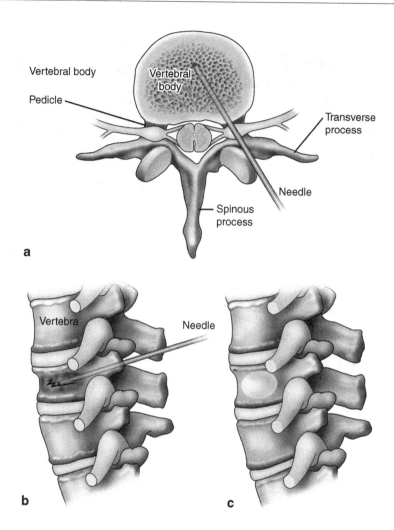

Fig. 5.5 (a–c) Lumbar vertebral body. Transpedicular needle placement

Percutaneous vertebroplasty was pioneered by the interventional neuroradiologist Herve Deramond in 1984. This involves the transpedicular (or lateral) introduction of a trocar needle into the compressed vertebral body using image guidance [10]. See Fig. 5.5a–c.

The mechanism of back pain associated with vertebral compression fractures is not completely understood, yet the leading school of thought revolves around vertebral fracture fragment mobility. Cement fixation not only provides solid mechanical and structural support, but also greatly reduces pain caused by fracture particles grinding across one another. See Fig. 5.6a–d.

Balloon kyphoplasty is closely related to vertebroplasty and indeed was initially coined "balloon-assisted vertebroplasty." First described in 2001 by Lieberman et al. [10], kyphoplasty primarily differs from vertebroplasty in the use of a pressurized balloon tamp to restore vertebral body height. The use of a balloon (tamp) and cement

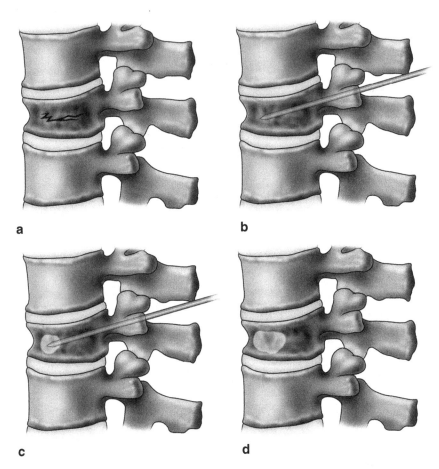

Fig. 5.6 (a) Compression fracture. (b) Trochar needle in place. (c) Cement filling. (d) Completion of vertebroplasty

injection results in decreased vertebral body deformity and possible height restoration. See Fig. 5.7a–d.

Like vertebroplasty, the primary aim of kyphoplasty is to provide pain relief from symptomatic vertebral compression fractures. Several studies have indicated that kyphoplasty and vertebroplasty provide equivalent pain relief [11]. However, due to vertebral body height restoration, kyphoplasty can theoretically provide the additional benefits of minimizing kyphotic appearance (i.e., the "dowager's hump") and kyphosis-related restrictive lung disease.

Contraindications for vertebroplasty and kyphoplasty are generally the same and include first and foremost the presence of infection or significant coagulopathy. The introduction of cement into an infected vertebral body would seed the fixation and further complicate a preexisting osteomyelitis and/or discitis. Patients with abnormal coagulation are at increased risk for local hematoma formation and mass effect on the spinal canal.

Other contraindications include bone cement allergy, unstable fractures involving the posterior vertebral body or spinal canal, inability to discern a specific anatomic level of

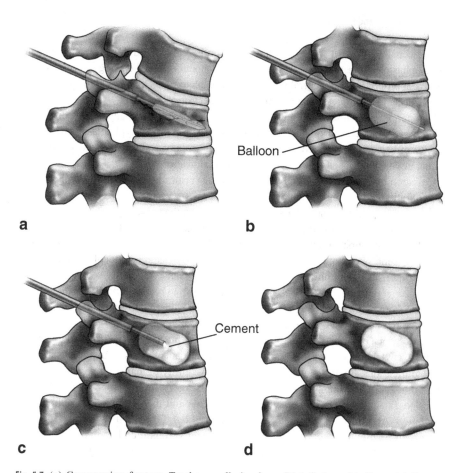

Fig. 5.7 (a) Compression fracture. Trochar needle in place. (b) Inflation of balloon. (c) Cement filling. (d) Completion of kyphoplasty

fracture, and improvement of symptoms with conservative management. It should be noted that percutaneous vertebral augmentations are currently *not* appropriate for painless, asymptomatic compression fractures [12].

Relative contraindications include vertebra plana, neurologic dysfunction caused by severe vertebral body destruction, symptomatic malignant involvement of the spinal nerves or spinal cord, and patient inability to remain prone and still for the procedure. Pregnancy is a relative contraindication, as the cement may have teratogenic effects.

Profoundly collapsed vertebrae without neural compromise, while technically challenging to approach and inject, are not a contraindication to vertebroplasty or kyphoplasty with studies having now described successful vertebroplasty in thoracolumbar burst fractures [13]. Caution is advised, since the presence of retropulsed fragments on pre-procedure imaging is also a relative contraindication; pieces can be pushed into the spinal canal and compress or damage the cord. See Fig. 5.4.

Consult, Consent, and Preparation

A brief consultation visit with the patient and family allows for a thorough and accurate history, physical exam, and review of imaging and laboratory data. Drawing screening blood work is appropriate. This generally includes a complete blood count (CBC), coagulation parameters, and a complete metabolic panel (e.g., electrolytes, etc).

In general, intravenous conscious sedation is used for vertebral body biopsy, disc aspiration, vertebroplasty, and kyphoplasty. Should a vertebroplasty or kyphoplasty be planned, absence of bacteremia or osteomyelitis of the spine must be confirmed. Injection of bone cement in this clinical setting is an absolute contraindication.

Cessation of anticoagulants and antiplatelet drugs prior to vertebroplasty, kyphoplasty, disc aspiration/biopsy, and vertebral body biopsy is appropriate.

Up to three or four levels of VCFs may be treated on the same day, but some operators and patients may wish to stage a series of procedures, starting with the most severely symptomatic sites first, and then assessing the patient's pain relief in the follow-up visit.

For consent, one should review the pre- and post-procedure protocol as well as the benefits and risks of complications with vertebroplasty and kyphoplasty.

Both vertebroplasty and kyphoplasty have been shown to be quite effective in alleviating back pain from VCFs with 90% of patients experiencing pain relief within days of the procedure. (See full discussion of data in the Outcomes section in this chapter.) Controversy does exist as to which of these two procedures will better benefit a specific patient, and it may be helpful to cover these discrepancies in order to keep the patient's expectations realistic.

Complications are quite rare but include the possibility of inadvertent cement deposition into the neural canal, requiring additional surgery for decompression. Cement may also exit the vertebral body via draining veins and then embolize to pulmonary circulation. Additionally, there may be an increased risk for patients who have the spinal cement fixation procedure to develop subsequent vertebral body compression fractures at sites adjacent to the treated levels. (See full discussion of data in Complications section in this chapter.)

Technique

Equipment and Materials

Radiopaque Bone Cement

Medical grade polymer (cement) used in spine interventions is usually polymethylmethacrylate (PMMA). PMMA is an acrylic polymer that is supplied as a liquid monomer and powdered polymer. After the two components are mixed, a highly exothermic reaction follows with subsequent hardening [14]. An essential component to this mixture is the addition of a radiopaque material to allow visualization during fluoroscopically guided percutaneous delivery into the bone. The most commonly used opacifying agent is powdered barium, typically mixed as a 30% by volume component [14]. Tantalum, another radiopaque powder, is occasionally used. See Fig. 5.8a, b.

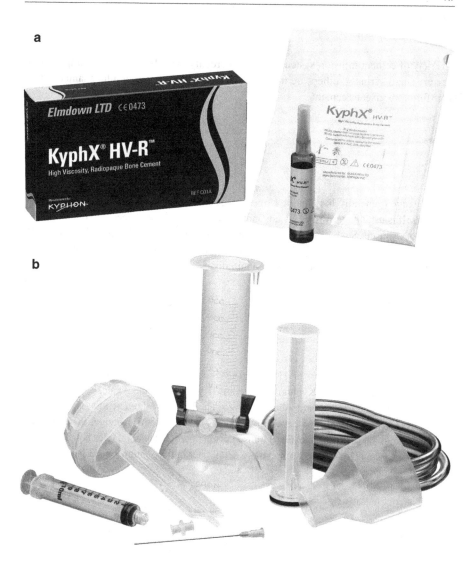

Fig. 5.8 (a) Kyphon® bone cement (Kyphon Inc, Sunnyvale, CA). (b) Kyphon® HV-R® (High Viscosity – Radiopaque) (Kyphon Inc, Sunnyvale, CA) bone cement and mixing system. It is essential to time the mixing of the cement to provide adequate "working time" (Courtesy of Medtronic, Inc. With permission)

Recently, new PMMA cements have been developed that contain a small amount (approximately 10%) of hydroxyapatite. These Food and Drug Administration (FDA) approved cements theoretically promote bone regeneration; however, large-scale studies have yet to prove this claim. Hydroxyapatite cements usually utilize the same mixing and infusion systems, and possess the same "working times" before they become too hard to infuse into the vertebral body.

Cement Infusion Systems

A variety of cement infusion systems are commercially available. Some are simple, high pressure small syringes; others are more elaborate screw type or hydraulic chambers, the latter for more viscous cement.

Needles

Vertebroplasty

Eleven gauge (generally lumbar) or 13 gauge (generally thoracic) needles are used. The biopsy itself is usually performed by advancing a coaxially directed needle to obtain a core of bone or aspirate. Such needle tips are serrated (cutting) or beveled and very sharp. If there is no suspicion of osteomyelitis, the operator may proceed to vertebroplasty without removing the transpedicular needle placed initially.

Needles

Kyphoplasty

Nine gauge (generally lumbar) or 11 gauge (generally thoracic) diamond tip or spade tip needles are usually used. The Kyphon® lumbar kits (Kyphon Inc, Sunnyvale, CA) come with one diamond tip and one spade tip, both 9 gauge. The Kyphon® thoracic kits (Kyphon Inc, Sunnyvale, CA) come with one bevel tip and one spade tip, both 11 gauge. Such needles allow entry into the vertebral body via a transpedicular, parapedicular, or occasionally posterolateral approach. (This is discussed in more detail later in this section.) See Fig. 5.9a–c.

Balloon Tamp: Kyphoplasty

These high-pressure balloons vary in size. Kyphon® (Kyphon Inc, Sunnyvale, CA) offers kits with 20 mm by 3 cm, 15 mm by 2 cm, 10 mm by 2 cm, and 15 mm by 3 cm balloons. See Fig. 5.10a–c.

Bone Biopsy Devices and Drills

A variety of devices are commercially available depending on the manufacturer. These are generally advanced coaxially through the transpedicular needle after the stylet is removed. Core samples are usually sent for either culture, surgical pathology, or both depending on the clinical concerns (e.g., metastatic disease, primary bone tumors such as multiple myeloma, suspected infection, etc.). To supplement the creation of a channel after bone biopsy, drills may be used to further create space for the balloon tamp. (Note: Vertebroplasty and kyphoplasty are absolutely contraindicated in a patient with suspected vertebral body osteomyelitis.)

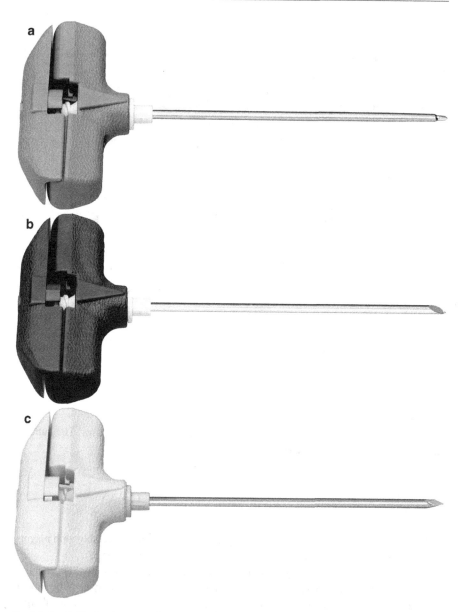

Fig. 5.9 (**a–c**) Kyphoplasty needles come in a variety of different tips used according to the operator's preference. (**a**) The green needle is a diamond tip. (**b**) The blue needle is a bevel or "spade" tip. (**c**) The white needle is a trocar tip (Courtesy of Medtronic, Inc. With permission)

Vertebroplasty or Kyphoplasty Kits

Depending on the manufacturer, a complete kit or tray with optional accessories is available and serves to meet the needs of a variety of practitioners.

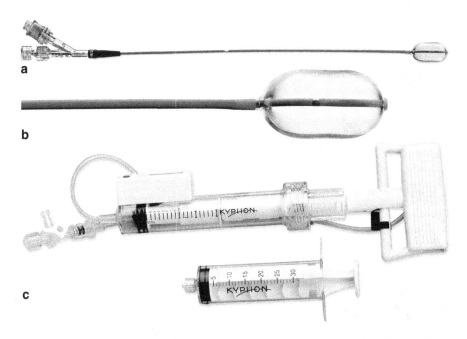

Fig. 5.10 (a–c) The balloon and inflation system used in kyphoplasty. (a) Balloon catheter. (b) Balloon inflated. (c) Inflation syringe (Courtesy of Medtronic, Inc. With permission)

Contrast

Contrast is generally used to opacify the balloon in kyphoplasty procedures. The authors prefer Isovue-M®200 (Bracco Diagnostics Inc, Princeton, NJ).

Procedure Start

Biplanar imaging is extremely useful in visualization of the spine, preferably with magnification options. Conscious sedation is administered (or anesthesia support).

Prophylactic IV antibiotic administration for the patient against skin flora is generally recommended for vertebral augmentation procedures. The authors usually give the patient a single dose of cefazolin 1 g intravenous at the procedure start, unless there is an allergy. Early practitioners of vertebroplasty added gentamicin or tobramycin to the cement mixture as prophylaxis against infection. However, Kallmes reports that tobramycin may markedly alter the viscosity of the PMMA mixture, resulting in diminished cement "working time" [14].

The patient is placed prone. The hips are slightly elevated for patient comfort. The arms are tucked forward under the patient's head or neck region to avoid obstruction on the lateral fluoroscopic imaging (Fig. 5.11a, b). Some operators may prefer to have the patient on the side. The appropriate vertebral body level is localized, and digital spot images are

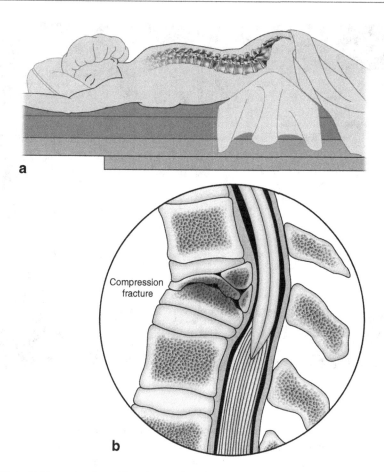

Fig. 5.11 (**a, b**) The patient is positioned prone for spinal augmentation. The arms are placed above the patient in order to allow for an unobstructed view during lateral fluoroscopy

obtained (scout images). Once the specific spinal level is marked, the overlying skin site is prepped and draped in the usual sterile fashion.

Step by Step

Balloon Kyphoplasty

Depending on the extent of disease in the vertebral biopsy, a unilateral or bilateral transpedicular access is chosen. For example, in the setting of metastatic disease found in the lateral half of the vertebral body, a unipedicular access may be sufficient (i.e., accessing the vertebral body from a single pedicle on the side with disease). In contrast, disease (i.e., fracture or tumor involving the entire vertebral body) may require use of a bilateral approach.

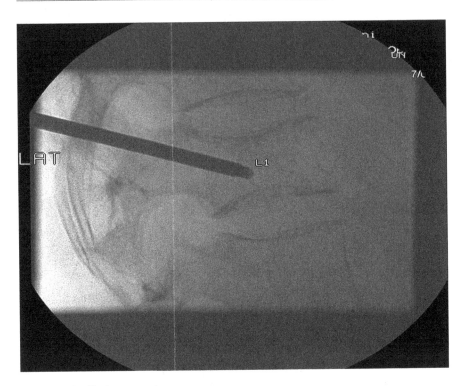

Fig. 5.12 Unipedicular approach

Although there are several commercially available kits, the authors use the Kyphon® set (Kyphon Inc, Sunnyvale, CA). Depending on the level (i.e., lumbar or thoracic), the needle size (gauge) varies (i.e., 11 gauge for thoracic, 9 gauge for lumbar).

In the anterior–posterior (AP) projection, the pedicles are visualized using magnification mode. On the oval of the pedicle on the patient's left side, the 9 o'clock position is chosen. Local anesthetic is administered (i.e., skin, subcutaneous tissue, muscle, and periosteum). After a skin nick with a #11 blade, the needle is advanced under biplane fluoroscopic guidance (Fig. 5.12). Care is taken to avoid transgressing both the medial and inferior aspects of the pedicle. This will prevent inadvertent injury to the thecal sac and neural canal (i.e., medially) and the nerve root that exits under the pedicle (i.e., inferior). Thus, the "upper-outer quadrant" of the pedicle is generally safe. In patients with absent (i.e., destroyed) pedicles, a parapedicular or occasionally a posterolateral approach may be required.

The needle tip may be "diamond" tip, "bevel" tip, or "trocar" tip depending on operator preference. Once the needle is angled and advanced through the pedicle, the stylet is removed. A bone biopsy device is then advanced coaxially and, with careful rotation by hand, the biopsy device is advanced through the vertebral body until a core is obtained. Lateral fluoroscopy is critical in monitoring this maneuver. The biopsy device (with bone core) is removed, and the bone sample is retrieved. This is sent for analysis, generally to surgical pathology and, if appropriate, microbiology for culture.

After bone biopsy, a small rotational hand drill may be used to create a further channel for placement of the balloon tamp (balloon). If bilateral (i.e., bilateral transpedicular)

Fig. 5.13 (a, b) Kyphoplasty.
(a) Lumbar spine. **(b)**
Thoracic spine

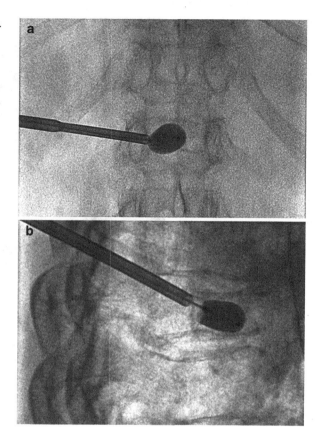

access is required, the same procedure is repeated on the opposite pedicle. In this example, having placed both balloon tamps, attention is directed to the mixing of "bone cement" (cyanoacrylate). This is accomplished according to the manufacturer's directions. See Fig. 5.13a, b.

Depending on the manufacturer, the cement sets up (hardens) rather quickly. Therefore, efficient work is required. While the cement is being loaded in the bone fillers, the balloon tamps are inflated with iodinated contrast to create a space in the compressed vertebral body (maximum inflation is 400 lb/in.^{2}). Biplane fluoroscopy is used. Care is taken to avoid over inflation so as not to break through the vertebral body end plate or into other adjacent structures (e.g., neural canal). See Fig. 5.14.

After balloon-tamp inflation, the balloons are sequentially deflated and removed from the needles. The bone fillers are advanced, and radiopaque cement is pushed into the vertebral body cavity, filling the void created by the balloon tamp. This step must be monitored with fluoroscopy so that the cement (a) is not injected to a point where it tracks back into the neural canal and (b) does not track across the vertebral body end plate into the disc space or other paravertebral body structures (e.g., veins, etc). The use of magnification views and careful AP, lateral, and occasionally oblique fluoroscopic monitoring during bone cement injection cannot be overemphasized. See Fig. 5.15.

Fig. 5.14 The cement is mixed and loaded

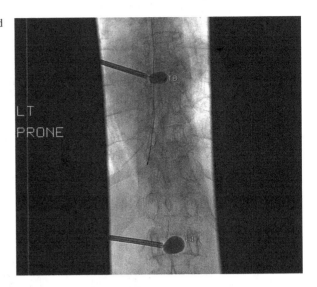

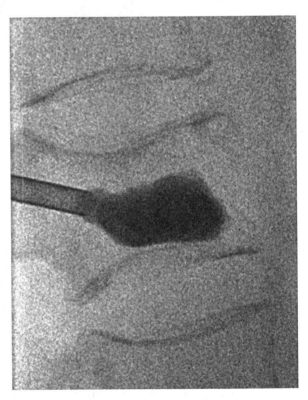

Fig. 5.15 Lateral lumbar spine. A magnification view is best to monitor progress during cement injection

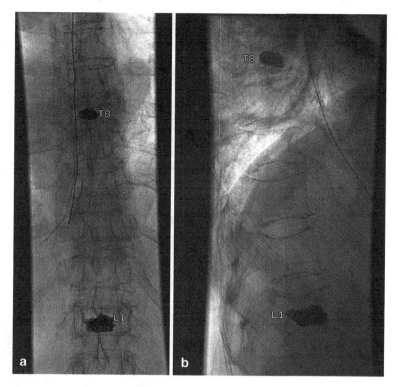

Fig. 5.16 (**a, b**) AP and lateral lumbar spine views. Completion of kyphoplasty

After installation of cement via the needles placed transpedicular, the cement is "tapped" in place to prevent cement "tails" from being pulled inadvertently back into the soft tissues of the back. Should this occur, the cement hardens and may cause future discomfort (i.e., a soft tissue foreign body).

The last step is to remove the cannulas and to apply pressure to the puncture sites. After achieving hemostasis, small pressure dressings are applied. Some operators will close the skin "stab" incision with steri-strips. Alternatively, others utilize tissue adhesive (Dermabond®, Ethicon Inc., Somerville, NJ). See Fig. 5.16a, b.

Newer developments include the use of directional balloons that allow (a) a unipedicular approach and (b) the ability to rotate the balloon tamp so it reaches the center of the vertebral body (e.g., Kyphon® Kyphx® Exact and Elevate™ balloons, Kyphon Inc, Sunnyvale, CA).

Vertebroplasty

The technique for vertebroplasty is similar to that of kyphoplasty except no balloon tamp is used. The patient preparation, anatomic approach, materials, and post-procedure care are the same. The needle size is smaller, generally 11 gauge for lumbar and 13 gauge for thoracic vertebral bodies. The PMMA is generally less viscous. See Fig. 5.17a–d. Vertebroplasty is preferred in the setting of severe compression fracture (i.e., vertebra plana).

Fig. 5.17 (**a–d**) Vertebroplasty

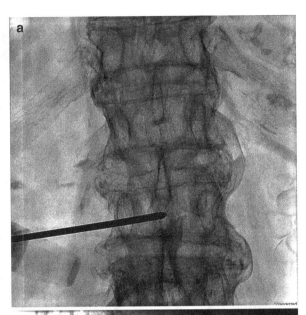

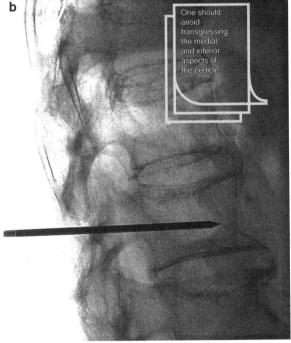

One should
avoid
transgressing
the medial
and inferior
aspects of
the pedicle

Fig. 5.17 (continued)

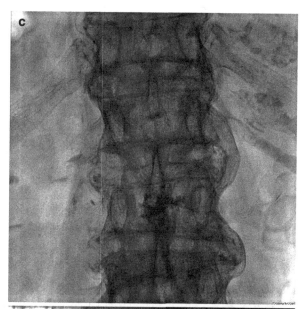

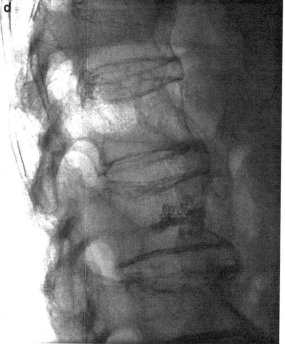

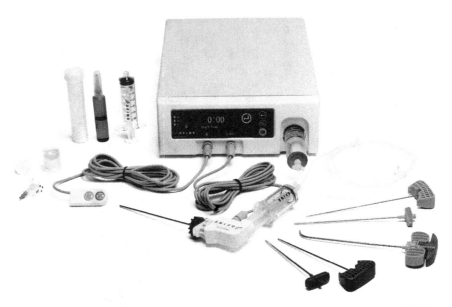

Fig. 5.18 Radiofrequency kyphoplasty kit (StabiliT™ vertebral augmentation system, DFINE, Inc., San Jose, CA) (Courtesy of DFINE, Inc. With permission)

Radiofrequency Kyphoplasty: Overview and Technique

Recent developments in the field of vertebral augmentation include Radio Frequency Kyphoplasty (RFK) (StabiliT™ Vertebral Augmentation System, DFINE Inc, San Jose, CA). As with kyphoplasty, access to the vertebral body is obtained under fluoroscopic or CT guidance through a transpedicular approach. This system has several key differences that set it apart from conventional balloon kyphoplasty. See Fig. 5.18.

Instead of using a balloon to create a cavity for injection of PMMA, a curved articulating osteotome is inserted through the needle canula and is used to create a cavity in the vertebral body. The size and location of the created cavity can be tailored to the patient by varying the angulation of the osteotome and the number of passes through the vertebrae. After the cavity is created, a proprietary ultra-high viscosity formulation of PMMA bone cement is injected through the canula via a specialized hydraulic delivery system.

The term "RF Kyphoplasty" comes from the radiofrequency energy, which is continuously applied to the cement by the delivery system just prior to infusion into the vertebral body and begins the curing process and further increases the viscosity of the cement. Under fluoroscopic observation, the cement mixture is slowly injected through the delivery cannula using a hydraulic pump located in the control unit. One of the advantages of this technique is that the delivery of cement via the hydraulic pump allows the operator to stand up to 10 ft away from the patient and operate the system via a remote control unit, thus significantly reducing radiation exposure to the operator. The amount of RF energy applied to the cement is automatically varied by the control unit throughout the procedure to maintain a relatively stable viscosity while providing a prolonged "working time" of approximately 30 min. The system is 10 gauge and can be used in both thoracic and lumbar spine.

Hints, Technical Points, Pitfalls, and Pearls

For vertebroplasty or kyphoplasty, an orthopedic bone mallet may occasionally be needed to advance the needle through the pedicle. This may be especially true in a young patient with dense bone (e.g., in the setting of a compressed fracture sustained in trauma). Patients with osteoporotic compression fractures or metastatic disease rarely require the use of a mallet. The bone is often soft enough to advance the needle with gentle forward force and rotation of the hub.

For thoracic vertebral body balloon kyphoplasty, a 13 gauge needle is used given the smaller diameter of the thoracic pedicles. For thoracic pedicle access, transpedicular access is more vertically oriented as compared to a lumbar transpedicular access. The lumbar access has the hub of the needle oriented more lateral with the tip coursing medial.

With kyphoplasty, depending on the severity of the compression fracture, vertebral body height augmentation may be minimal. Despite this, significant pain relief is often achieved even in the setting of bony destruction (e.g., metastatic disease).

The presence of cyanoacrylate (cement) does not prevent further therapy such as systemic chemotherapy or radiation therapy (i.e., in malignant disease).

Occasionally, in the setting of bony destruction, a bone biopsy may initially be performed. Later, when cultures or pathology results are back, the vertebroplasty or kyphoplasty procedure may be completed if there is no evidence of osteomyelitis. If the initial transpedicular access has been appropriately chosen, the same access site through the pedicle may be used at the later date (e.g., several days to a week later). Should cement be deposited in infected bone, the resulting infection would prove extremely difficult if not impossible to treat (i.e., to sterilize). The patient could require surgery to remove infected bone and cement that has been colonized with bacteria.

Postoperative Care, Discharge Instructions, and Follow-Up

Once inside the vertebral body, the polymethylmethacrylate (bone cement) hardens quickly. By the time the procedure is completed, the cement has generally "set up." The patient may therefore be readily transferred and, if appropriate, the patient's head may be elevated slightly on the gurney (i.e., no need for the patient to remain absolutely "flat").

The patient is removed to a stretcher and monitored for a few hours in the recovery room, depending on the amount of sedation given. Vertebral body augmentation procedures are generally performed on an outpatient basis. If the patient is in poor health, overnight "short stay" admission is reasonable.

The patient may ambulate when safe to do so. Some operators will restrict patient activity to bed rest for a few hours after the procedure to assure theoretical cement setting and spine stabilization prior to ambulation.

Generally, ibuprofen or other nonsteroidal anti-inflammatory medication is all that is required for pain management. Occasionally, a stronger analgesic is required. The authors have found that initial application of an ice pack, later followed by heat (i.e., heating pad), is helpful (i.e., the sites are treated like a musculoskeletal injury or "sprain").

Outcomes

Vertebroplasty

Studies have proven that vertebroplasty is highly successful in reducing pain associated with compression fractures. According to most studies, over 90% of patients with osteoporotic VCFs who underwent vertebroplasty experienced at least some pain relief as demonstrated by an 11-point Visual Analog Scale (VAS) comparing pre- and post-procedural pain. The majority of one level vertebroplasty patients report this pain relief within 48–72 h post-procedure, while multilevel patients require a longer amount of time to experience pain relief. Studies have attempted to quantify this pain relief, one of which states that patients experience a 57% decrease in pain at a follow-up time of 2 weeks [15]. Others demonstrate a VAS pain decrease averaging 6 points, usually from a VAS of approximately 8 to a VAS of 2. Patients with less common causes of VCFs such as malignancy, trauma, myeloma, and angioma demonstrate similar results [1, 2, 16].

Do et al. reported a series of patients with painful osteoporotic vertebral body fractures who were randomized to either undergo vertebroplasty or 6 weeks of continued medical therapy, followed by vertebroplasty if needed. The analysis showed marked improvement in the treatment group (vertebroplasty), but no improvement in the medical therapy group. In the medical treatment arm, vertebroplasty was offered after the 6 week medical trial, and, in most cases, vertebroplasty relieved pain that medical therapy could not [17].

Another benefit to vertebral augmentation following fracture is an increase in respiratory function. Tanigawa et al. performed vertebroplasty on 99 patients (88 of whom were women, mean age 74) and evaluated respiratory function with the use of a spirometer. Percent vital capacity (%VC), percent forced vital capacity (%FVC), and percent forced expiratory volume in 1 s (FEV1.0%) were measured before, 1 day after, and 1 month after the procedure. Statistically significant increases in mean %VC and %FVC were noted 1 month post-vertebroplasty; however, no differences were seen the day after the procedure [18]. Respiratory function results post-kyphoplasty are thought to mirror those mentioned here.

Kyphoplasty

Balloon kyphoplasty patients experience similar pain relief to those who have undergone vertebroplasty. The "mechanical consolidation" provided by the bone cement functions identically in kyphoplasty as it does in vertebroplasty. The major debate surrounding kyphoplasty is the concept of height restoration [1].

A 2005 Majd et al. study found 89% of patients experience pain relief by first follow-up (range 6–36 months, mean 21 months). The remaining patients had persistent pain and were diagnosed with either degenerative disc disease or a new fracture. In fact, 12% of the patients in this particular study eventually needed an additional kyphoplasty procedure to treat new, symptomatic fractures [11].

Lane et al. have demonstrated an average height restoration of 3.7 mm in the anterior vertebral body, 4.7 mm in the mid-vertebral body, and 1.5 mm in the posterior vertebral body. Supporting studies have concluded that approximately 70% (69%) of fractures treated with kyphoplasty result in a mean midline restoration of 50% of lost vertebral height, while average anterior vertebral height restoration is 30% in only 63% of fractures [11, 19].

Conversely, many believe that vertebral height restoration from kyphoplasty is minimal and that patients who have undergone vertebroplasty are just as likely to experience the same kyphotic correction as they are more likely to improve their posture with less spine pain [20]. To date, no studies have consistently proven any significant association with improvement of vertebral height/kyphotic angle and pain relief [21].

At the time of this publication, no large studies directly comparing RF kyphoplasty (RFK) with kyphoplasty or vertebroplasty have been published in the United States. Abstracts for two studies out of Germany recently presented at the 2010 International Osteoporosis Foundation meeting suggest that early experience with RFK demonstrates advantages over vertebroplasty [22, 23]. One study compared 60 patients treated with RFK to a control group of 39 patients treated with vertebroplasty, and found a significantly decreased incidence of cement leakage (5.4% in the RFK group versus 59.6% in the control group, a 91% decrease), with no incidence of symptomatic cement leakage in the RFK group [22]. Another study by the same author followed 63 patients after an RFK procedure and found a 4.4% cement leakage rate, all asymptomatic [23]. Early data suggest that the increased viscosity of the PMMA formulation used during RFK offers a decrease in the rate of cement extravasation, while still offering the clinical benefits associated with conventional methods of spine augmentation. More studies clearly need to be performed, particularly comparing the safety and effectiveness of RFK to Balloon Kyphoplasty.

It is widely accepted that both vertebroplasty and kyphoplasty are superior to medical management in the palliative treatment of symptomatic osteoporotic VCFs. With either procedure, if there is indeed no pain relief or improvement of pain symptoms, one should investigate other spinal levels for acute fracture and/or other etiologies as the source of pain (e.g., soft tissue injury, degenerative disc disease, etc.).

Controversy over Outcomes

In August 2009, two well-publicized articles by Kallmes et al. and Buchbinder et al. were published in the *The New England Journal of Medicine*, concluding that a control group sham procedure resulted in similar pain and pain-related disability improvements when compared to vertebroplasty on patients with osteoporotic vertebral compression fractures [24]. Buchbinder et al. went on to say that when compared to a sham procedure, vertebroplasty provides no added benefit to patients with osteoporotic vertebral compression fractures at 1 week, or 1, 3, or 6 months post-procedure [25].

In the multicenter study by Kallmes et al., 131 patients with 1–3 osteoporotic VCFs each were randomly assigned to undergo either vertebroplasty or a sham (control) procedure. Both procedures involved subcutaneous numbing with 1% lidocaine and periosteal infiltration of the pedicle(s) with 0.25% bupivacaine. Patients were then either assigned to the vertebroplasty group, or the control group in which neither PMMA cement nor needle were introduced, but pressure was put on the patient's back, a methacrylate monomer was opened to induce the smell of bone cement, and the patients were placed in the supine position post-intervention for 1–2 h before being discharged [24].

After the 68 vertebroplasties and 63 simulated procedures were performed, pain rating and disability scores were not significantly different at 1 month follow-up. Both groups experienced similar, immediate improvement in pain and disability scores. However, each patient was given the opportunity to switch groups after 1 month post-initial procedure if their pain relief was not adequate. At 3 months, 43% of the control group had decided to have vertebroplasty, while 12% of the vertebroplasty group opted to try the sham procedure [24].

Another trial by Buchbinder et al. involved randomly assigning patients with 1 or 2 osteoporotic VCFs less than 12 months old to vertebroplasty or a sham procedure. This trial's sham procedure was similar to that of Kallmes et al. Yet, practitioners actually introduced at 13 gauge needle and rested it on the lamina. The sharp stylet of a trocar needle was replaced with a blunt stylet, and the vertebral body was gently tapped to simulate vertebroplasty. PMMA was also prepared to fill the room with the distinct smell [25].

Pain at night and at rest, physical functioning, quality of life, and perceived improvement were all measured after 1 week, 1 month, 3 months, and 6 months post-intervention and compared to pre-procedure ratings. While both study groups experienced significant reductions in overall pain, vertebroplasty did not provide any statistically significant added benefit in any of the measured arenas [25].

In the months following these articles, vertebroplasty procedure numbers fell throughout the country. Given that balloon kyphoplasty is essentially "balloon-assisted vertebroplasty," it was no wonder that kyphoplasty use in the United States fell approximately 40% in the wake of the publication.

Soon thereafter, the Society of Interventional Radiology (SIR) and the *Journal of NeuroInterventional Surgery* both posted and published responses in the latter months of 2009. Citing the discordance of results from the majority of literature on vertebroplasty, as well as most practicing physicians' experiences, SIR applauded the efforts, yet scrutinized the study designs of both trials.

SIR believes that selection bias was introduced into the Kallmes et al. study as it screened 1,813 patients and excluded 1,682 for a variety of reasons. This left the trial with 131 patients (68 in the vertebroplasty group and 63 in the control group), while the study had initially called for 250. Also, screening bone scans and/or MRIs were not required for known fractures under 1 year of age. SIR stated that the small sample size could have had the potential to escape randomization and, therefore, it is not impossible that patients who had healed their VCF and thus had another cause for their acute pain were concentrated in the vertebroplasty group. In addition, SIR pointed out the large crossover rate discrepancy between those patients who received the sham procedure and wanted vertebroplasty (43%) and vice versa (12%) [26].

In regards to the Buchbinder et al. study, SIR commented on how out of 219 eligible patients, Buchbinder and colleagues only chose 78 to be enrolled, suggesting selection bias. Sixty-seven percent of the patients in the Buchbinder et al. study came from a single site and were performed by a single radiologist. Negative bias against vertebroplasty could have resulted if the single site and physician performing the interventions were more likely to provide conservative treatment. Lastly, the average volume of PMMA injected into the vertebrae in the Buchbinder et al. trial was 2.8 ml. This amount is significantly lower than that of other trials and may have contributed to the results [26].

The Journal of NeuroInterventional Surgery also criticized both study designs and was quick to point out that *The New England Journal of Medicine* created a media frenzy by publishing these two articles in the midst of a nationwide debate on health care reform and the costs associated with technologically advanced care [27].

Cost

Cost cannot be ignored in a discussion of vertebroplasty and kyphoplasty, as significant differences exist. Kyphoplasty kits cost approximately $3,500. The bone cement not included in the kit is another $175, putting the total device cost of kyphoplasty at around $3,675. Vertebroplasty trays, on the other hand, cost approximately $400. When the cost of bone cement is added in, vertebroplasty is approximately six times less expensive than kyphoplasty, and this only takes into account the equipment needed for each procedure. Another important factor in cost is whether the patient is undergoing conscious sedation or general anesthesia. While this decision should be patient based rather than procedure based, many kyphoplasties are performed in operating rooms with general anesthesia, and the patients are monitored overnight in the hospital. Some estimate that all of these differences summate to make kyphoplasty up to 10–20 times more costly than vertebroplasty [28]. Other considerations include the additional fluoroscopy time and procedure time associated with kyphoplasty that could be tying up the interventional radiology suite or operating room.

Complications

Complications associated with vertebroplasty and kyphoplasty, while rare, range from completely asymptomatic to life-threatening. The most significant complication is that of inadvertent cement deposition into the neural canal (e.g., epidural space, causing a fixed cord compression). This requires emergent surgical decompression. Another significant complication is that of inadvertent embolization of cement which, during placement, exits the vertebral body via draining veins. The cement may then embolize to pulmonary circulation.

In general, no more than three or four levels should be treated in a single setting. Case reports have appeared in which multiple levels (e.g., eight levels) have resulted in patient death. In some cases, pathologic analysis of the lungs at autopsy showed extensive fat emboli.

One study conducted on 880 patients (675 of which were female, with a mean age of 70 years) who underwent vertebroplasty reported asymptomatic venous PMMA leakage in over one third of patients, PMMA leakage into the disc in 15.5% of patients, asymptomatic PMMA lung embolism in 1.6% of patients, and nerve root irritation in 0.7% of patients [2]. By these estimates, approximately half of treated patients will experience some sort of minor complication, the majority of which are asymptomatic.

A comparative systematic review and meta-regression analysis of vertebroplasty and kyphoplasty procedures between 1980 and 2004 by Taylor et al. found a significantly higher rate of cement extravasations during vertebroplasty (40%) than kyphoplasty (8%). In addition, 3% of cement leaks during vertebroplasty were symptomatic, while none of the analyzed kyphoplasties resulted in symptomatic leaks [21]. Kyphoplasty proponents claim that creating a cavity within the vertebrae by inflating a balloon gives the cement a place to go and subsequently decreases the pressure created by injecting cement. This lower pressure upon cement injection leads to less cement extravasation outside the vertebral body. However, this same Taylor et al. study demonstrated that kyphoplasty patients experienced more total and adjacent post-procedure vertebral compression fractures than vertebroplasty patients [21].

There is a growing concern that vertebroplasty/kyphoplasty could increase the risk of subsequent vertebral body compression fractures at sites adjacent to treated levels. Series have been published documenting the incidence of new onset fractures following vertebroplasty, with most series showing approximately 20% incidences of new fractures within 1 year of the procedures. The majority of new fractures are adjacent to treated levels, suggesting a relationship between cemented vertebral bodies and new fracture events. However, it is also known that even in the absence of vertebroplasty, osteoporotic fractures tend to "cluster" in the mid-thoracic region and the thoracolumbar region [14]. In fact, an Anselmetti et al. study on 884 patients, of whom 750 were female (73.1%), over 5 years concluded that over two-thirds of VCFs occur between the levels on T11 and L2 [29]. Thus, adjacent level fractures may be expected. Given all this, systemic osteoporotic therapies should be instituted.

Summary and Conclusions

Spinal augmentation procedures are of proven benefit to symptomatic patients with back pain from compression fractures. While operators should be aware of the technical differences of the vertebroplasty and kyphoplasty procedures, there are important advantages and disadvantages specific to each method. The technical success rates for both procedures are comparable and quite high. Additionally, it appears that vertebroplasty may be less expensive than kyphoplasty. While serious complications following spinal augmentation are rare, an understanding of possible problems is paramount to the physicians when consulting and selecting patients. With appropriate clinical work-up and technique, spinal augmentation procedures are an invaluable and safe solution for symptomatic patients, providing durable pain relief for acute compression fractures.

References

1. Anselmetti GC, Muto M, Guglielmi G, Masal S. Percutaneous vertebroplasty or kyphoplasty. Radiol Clin North Am. 2010;48(3):641–9.
2. Anselmetti GC, Masala S, Manca A, Russo F, Eminefendic H, Regge D. Percutaneous vertebroplasty: 4 years experience on 880 consecutive patients [abstract]. SIR (Suppl). 2007;201:S75.
3. Coleman RE, Rubens RD. The clinical course of bone metastases from breast cancer. Br J Cancer. 1987;55:61.
4. Mundy GR. Metastasis to bone: causes, consequences and therapeutic opportunities. Nat Rev Cancer. 2002;2:584.
5. Chiang AC, Massague J. Molecular basis of metastasis. N Engl J Med. 2008;359:2814.
6. Coleman RE, Seamen JJ. The role of zolendronic acid in cancer: clinical studies in the treatment and prevention of bone metastases. Semin Oncol. 2001;28:11.
7. Stallmeyer MJB, Zoarski GH, Obuchowski AM. Optimizing patient. Selection in percutaneous vertebroplasty. J Vasc Interv Radiol. 2003;14(6):683–96.
8. Anselmetti GC, Manca A, Chiara G, Iussich G, Isaia G, Regge D. Percutaneous vertebroplasty in the osteoporotic patients: optimal indications and patient selection to improve clinical outcome. Personal experience in 1542 patients over 7 years [abstract]. SIR (Suppl). 2010;16:S8.
9. Philips FM. Minimally invasive treatments of osteoporotic vertebral compression fractures. Spine J. 2003;28(Suppl):45–52.
10. Lieberman IH, Dudeney S, Reinhardt MK, Bell G. Initial outcome and efficacy of "kyphoplasty" in the treatment of painful osteoporotic vertebral compression fractures. Spine (Phila Pa 1976). 2001;26:1631–8.
11. Majd ME, Farley S, Holt RT. Preliminary outcomes and efficacy of the first 360 consecutive kyphoplasties for the treatment of painful osteoporotic vertebral compression fractures. Spine J. 2005;5(3):244–55.
12. Denaro L, Longo UM, Denaro V. Vertebroplasty and kyphoplasty: reasons for concern? Orthop Clin North Am. 2009;40:465–71.
13. Cho DY, Lee WY, Sheu PC. Treatment of thoracolumbar burst fractures with polymethyl methacrylate vertebroplasty and short-segment pedicle screw fixation. Neurosurgery. 2003;53:1354–60, discussion 1360–1351.
14. Kallmes DF. Compression fractures: vertebroplasty. In: Siskin GP, editor. Interventional radiology in women's health. New York: Thieme Medical Publishers; 2009. p. 176–82.
15. Miller MJ. Efficacy and safety of percutaneous vertebroplasty in the treatment of osteoporotic compression fractures [abstract]. SIR (Suppl). 2007;204:S76.
16. Mcgirt MJ, Parker SL, Wolinsky JP, et al. Vertebroplasty and kyphoplasty for the treatment of vertebral compression fractures: an evidence-based review of the literature. Spine J. 2009;9(6):501–8.
17. Do HM, Kim BS, Marcellus ML, Curtis L, Marks MP. Prospective analysis of clinical outcomes after percutaneous vertebroplasty for painful osteoporotic vertebral body fractures. AJNR Am J Neuroradiol. 2005;26(7):1623–8.
18. Tanigawa N, Kariya S, Tokuda T, Nakatani M, Yagi R, Komemushi A, et al. Prospective analysis of respiratory function following percutaneous vertebroplasty for osteoporotic compression fractures [abstract]. SIR (Suppl). 2010;14:S8.
19. Lane JM, Girardi F, Paravaianen H, et al. Preliminary outcomes of the first 226 consecutive kyphoplasties for the fixation of painful osteoporotic vertebral compression fractures. Osteoporosis Int (Suppl). 2000;11:S206.
20. Mathis JM. Percutaneous vertebroplasty: complication avoidance and technique optimization. AJNR Am J Neuroradiol. 2003;24:1697–706.
21. Taylor RS, Taylor RJ, Fritzell P. Balloon kyphoplasty and vertebroplasty for vertebral compression fractures. Spine J. 2006;31(23):2747–55.

22. Pflugmacher R, Randau T, Kabir K, Wirtz DC. Radiofrequency (RF) kyphoplasty in comparison to vertebroplasty (VP): a prospective evaluation [abstract]. IOF World Congress on Osteoporosis, Florence, Italy. May 5–8, 2010.

23. Pflugmacher R, Randau T, Kabir K, Wirtz DC. Radiofrequency (RF) kyphoplasty in the treatment of osteolytic vertebral fractures [abstract]. IOF World Congress on Osteoporosis, Florence, Italy. May 5–8, 2010.

24. Kallmes DF et al. A randomized trial of vertebroplasty for osteoporotic spinal fractures. N Engl J Med. 2009;361(6):569–79.

25. Buchbinder R et al. Randomized trial of vertebroplasty for painful osteoporotic vertebral fractures. N Engl J Med. 2009;361(6):569–79.

26. Society of interventional radiology commentary on vertebroplasty and the August studies in the N Engl J Med. www.SIRweb.org. Accessed July 16, 2010.

27. Hirsch JA, Meyers PM, Jensen ME. P.S. augmentation. J Neurointerv Surg. 2009;1:179–80.

28. Mathis JM, Ortiz AO, Zoarski GH. Vertobroplasty versus kyphoplasty: a comparison and contrast. AJNR Am J Neuroradiol. 2004;25:840–5.

29. Anselmetti GC, Manca A, Russo F, Chiara G, Regge D. Percutaneous vertebroplasty in the osteoporotic patients: 5 years prospective follow-up in 884 consecutive patients [abstract]. SIR (Suppl). 2008;182:S69.

Spine Pain Management

Anthony C. Venbrux, Jozef M. Brozyna, Denis Primakov, and Wayne J. Olan

6

Introduction

The Center for Disease Control (CDC) publishes a report called the National Hospital Ambulatory Medical Care Survey every year. This report contains the top 10 reasons for Emergency Room (ER) visits, and, not surprisingly, back problems ranked number 3 for men and number 4 for women in the 15–64 age group [1]. Approximately 1,544,000 women went to the ER for their back problems, comprising 2.2% of all visits for all age groups, an alarmingly high rate. While back pain has epidemic proportions in the United States, the area continues to demonstrate some of the worst curative results in modern medicine. Alternative or adjuvant therapies for spinal back pain are in high demand. Traditionally treated by orthopedic surgeons and chiropractors, other medical specialties including Anesthesia, Rheumatology, and Interventional Radiology have joined the integrated effort to care for back pain, as a multidisciplinary approach is required to achieve any durable success.

Pathophysiology

Studies have reported that up to approximately 70% of people between the ages of 20 and 71 have experienced back pain. In addition, 55% of people within this age group have reported back pain within the last year. Lower back pain is by far the most common type of back pain, peaking at the age of 45. Women were more likely to report back pain in general, back pain in more than one area, as well as back pain for more days out of the year than men [2, 3].

Sixty percent of these patients will have chronic back pain that lasts at least 5 years after their initial episode, leaving this patient population with health, economic, and social problems that are not to be underestimated. Epidural steroid injections and nerve root injections are commonly used in pain management to minimize these problems.

A.C. Venbrux (✉)
Department of Radiology, Division of Interventional Radiology,
The George Washington University Medical Center, Washington, DC, USA
e-mail: avenbrux@mfa.gwu.edu

E.A. Ignacio and A.C. Venbrux (eds.), *Women's Health in Interventional Radiology*,
DOI 10.1007/978-1-4419-5876-1_6, © Springer Science+Business Media, LLC 2012

Epidural injections are more nonspecific and less localized, yet are typically effective in many patients with neck or back pain, spinal stenosis with neurogenic claudication, as well as radiculopathy. On the other hand, selective nerve blocks can provide diagnostic information, as well as deliver more steroids to a specifically targeted location to relieve nerve root irritation [4].

Clinical Manifestations

Patients will present with a widely varied clinical picture for back pain. Etiologies for low back pain are vast, and the specific pathologic process as well as the patient's overall health will dictate the quality and severity of the patient's back pain.

Anatomy

Anatomy of the Spine

Please refer to the Spine Anatomy section in Chap. 5.

Imaging

Most patients who seek pain management from Interventional Radiology have had the routine imaging for evaluation of the spine. Given the patient's constellation of symptoms, the Interventional Radiologist should be sure that the patient has had a reasonable investigation for other possible etiologies such as infection or malignancy, for which image-guided injection of analgesics or anti-inflammatories will do no good.

Radiographs or plain films of the spine are an economical screening tool and can be very helpful to localize the specific sites of bony degenerative change (e.g., compressing osteophytes).

Magnetic resonance imaging (MRI) is of course the gold standard for evaluation of the spine. Problems such as the presence of neuroforaminal narrowing from disc or bony degenerative change can be characterized in order to plan for nerve root interventions.

Patient Encounter

Indications and Contraindications

Nerve blocks, in comparison with epidural injections, are a more focal, localized approach to pain management. They are very useful in diagnosing which nerve is causing the patient's pain, as well as providing pain relief when the pain is stemming from a single nerve. Indications for nerve blocks include, but are not limited to, post-diskectomy patients with recurrent radiculopathy, disk herniation, subcostal pain from thoracic nerve roots, as well as diagnosing a specific nerve as the root of the patient's pain.

Contraindications include a history of allergy to the local anesthetics or steroids as well as coagulopathy [5].

Indications for epidural injections are similar to those for nerve blocks, but can be more helpful in instances in which pain cannot be localized to a single nerve. Indications for epidural injections include disk herniation, disk degeneration, spondylosis, pelvic pain, spinal stenosis, and radiculopathy.

Absolute contraindications to epidural injection are patient refusal, infection at the site, increased intracranial pressure, allergy to local anesthetics or steroids, and uncorrected hypovolemia. Relative contraindications include low platelet count, coagulopathy, and sepsis [6].

Consult, Consent, and Preparation

As with vertebroplasty and kyphoplasty, a brief consultation with the patient, reviews of history, physical exam, imaging, and laboratory results are necessary to confirm proper indication and exclude contraindications for the pain management procedure.

For nerve blocks, the authors prefer a platelet count of 60,000 or greater and an International Normalized Ratio (INR) no greater than 1.5. "Normal" values are obviously desired when possible. In general, discontinuation of antiplatelet medications is preferred but may not be possible. In these cases (e.g., in a patient who has received a drug-eluting coronary stent), the authors stop anticoagulants (e.g., unfractionated or low-molecular-weight heparin) but do not stop antiplatelet drugs.

In contrast, epidural injections generally require stricter coagulation parameters. If clinically possible, antiplatelet drugs are discontinued approximately 1 week before the procedure, and INR should be no greater than 1.2–1.5. Warfarin should also be discontinued 5–7 days prior to the procedure so that prothrombin time (PT) and INR are normal.

Patients may receive local anesthetic alone for nerve blocks (i.e., injection of steroid plus anesthetic) and epidural injections. If conscious sedation will be used, the patient will require adequate intravenous access.

Technique

Equipment and Materials

Needles

Twenty-one or 22 gauge spinal needles may be used both for injection of contrast to outline the nerve sheath (nerve block) or the epidural space (e.g., epidural injection).

Contrast

As previously noted, contrast is generally used to confirm spinal needle tip placement in pain management (i.e., nerve sheath outline during a "nerve block" or epidural space opacification during an epidural injection). The authors prefer Isovue-M®200 (Bracco Diagnostics Inc, Princeton, NJ) for nerve blocks/epidural injections.

Local Anesthesia

For nerve blocks, bupivacaine (Hospira Inc., Lake Forest, IL) 0.25% or 0.5% (preservative free) is generally preferred by the authors.

Steroids

The use of steroids varies. For lumbar or thoracic nerve blocks, the authors use methylprednisolone acetate (Depo-Medrol®, Pfizer Inc, New York, NY). Generally, 40 mg of the steroid plus 3–4 mls of 0.25% or 0.5% bupivacaine is injected. As mentioned earlier, methylprednisolone acetate "settles" in a syringe (i.e., particulate) and should be avoided for cervical nerve blocks. Instead, the authors use dexamethasone 12.5 mg in the cervical region. This liquid avoids potential risk for particulate embolization should the needle tip enter an arterial branch during a cervical nerve block. Some operators use triamcinolone as well [7].

Procedure Start

The goal of these image-guided procedures is pain relief. Generally, this consists of injection of contrast to confirm needle tip localization and injection of a longer acting anesthetic, coupled with an anti-inflammatory steroid. The procedures are performed on an outpatient basis and generally using only a local anesthetic. Verbal feedback from the patient is very helpful to determine the appropriate level of analgesia. This is especially true in patients with multilevel disc disease or severe degenerative disease (osteoarthritis).

Needle placement may be performed using high-resolution C-arm fluoroscopy, biplane fluoroscopy, or CT guidance.

Antibiotic administration is generally not required.

Step by Step

Lumbar Nerve Block

After informed consent, the patient is placed prone. The appropriate level is prepped and draped. If C-arm fluoroscopy is employed, the C-arm is rotated ipsilaterally so that the bony anatomy of the lumbar spine is visualized in an oblique projection, approximately 15–20°. If the patient has scoliosis or anatomic deformity, the angulation may change significantly.

After local anesthetic (superficial and deep), a 22 gauge needle is advanced such that the tip is positioned underneath the pedicle (Fig. 6.1a, b). On the lateral projection, the tip is advanced until it reaches the midpoint of the intervertebral foramen. The stylet is removed. No blood or cerebrospinal fluid (CSF) should be seen in the hub of the needle. If this is the case, the stylet is reintroduced and the needle tip is repositioned (generally slightly more lateral to the initial trajectory).

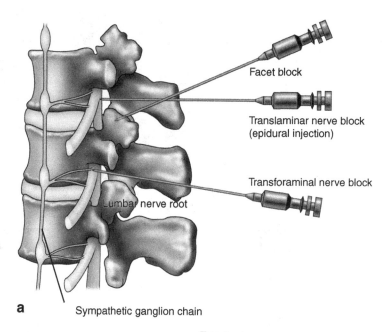

Facet block

Translaminar nerve block
(epidural injection)

Transforaminal nerve block

Lumbar nerve root

a   Sympathetic ganglion chain

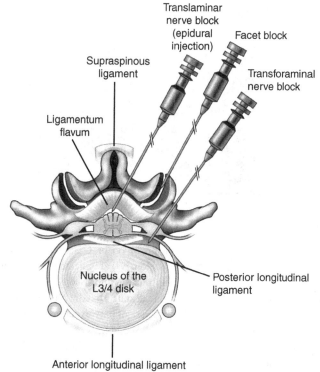

Translaminar
nerve block
(epidural
injection)   Facet block

Supraspinous
ligament   Transforaminal
nerve block

Ligamentum
flavum

Nucleus of the
L3/4 disk   Posterior longitudinal
ligament

b   Anterior longitudinal ligament

Fig. 6.1 (**a**, **b**) Various needle positions for injection at the spine

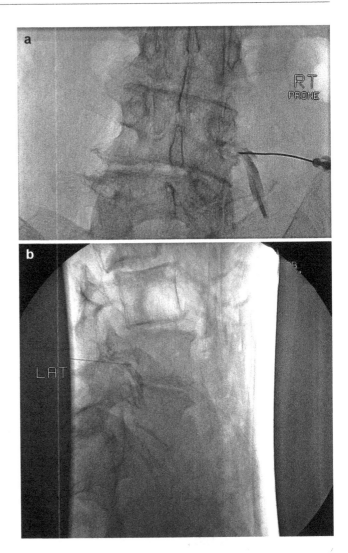

Having removed the stylet and finding no blood or CSF, approximately 0.5 ml of Isovue-M®200 (Bracco Diagnostics Inc, Princeton, NJ) are injected. This outlines the nerve sheath, a diagonal, inferolateral linear density seen on fluoroscopy. See Fig. 6.2a, b.

At this point, 40 mg of methylprednisolone acetate mixed with approximately 3–4 mls of 0.5% bupivacaine are injected slowly. The patient may experience transient pain in the appropriate nerve distribution (radiculopathy) or numbness or a combination of both. The patient may also experience temporary extremity muscle weakness, which may last several hours. The patient should be warned of this, lest there be a fall when beginning to ambulate. Some operators prefer 0.25% bupivacaine to lessen the chance of transient motor weakness.

Thoracic Nerve Block

With the patient prone, a posterolateral approach is used. After sterile skin preparation and appropriate draping, local anesthetic is injected in the skin and subcutaneous tissues. This is centered at the inferior aspect of the rib. A 21 gauge needle is advanced until the rib is felt; then the tip is "walked off" the rib until bone is no longer felt. The needle tip should suddenly advance deeper in the intercostal space. The needle can then be angulated slightly such that the tip is just under the inferior edge of the rib and adjacent to the neurovascular bundle, which runs along the inside inferior border of the rib. Oblique fluoroscopy will help determine depth, as advancing the needle too deep may result in a pneumothorax.

The stylet is removed. Approximately 0.5 ml of iodinated contrast are injected to be certain that the needle tip is not in the pleural space or lung parenchyma. If the needle tip is in the appropriate position, methylprednisolone acetate (80 mg) plus approximately 3 mls of 0.5% (or 0.25%) bupivacaine are injected. The needle is removed (Note: For thoracic nerve blocks, one may wish to inject one level above and below. This will eliminate the overlapping dermatome pain pattern. These other two locations receive bupivacaine only; the targeted site in between is injected with bupivacaine plus steroid).

Cervical Nerve Block

Cervical blocks are more technically challenging and therefore should probably be reserved for those operators who have more technical experience with spinal injections.

Serious neurologic and vascular complications can occur even when the procedure is performed according to accepted standard technique (See full discussion in Complications section in this chapter).

The patient is placed supine. An anterolateral approach is used. After sterile skin preparation and draping, the skin and subcutaneous tissues are anesthetized with a local anesthetic. A 25 gauge needle (21 gauge will suffice if 25 is not available) is advanced, and care is taken to avoid puncturing the carotid artery or jugular vein. After injecting contrast (Isovue-M®200, Bracco Diagnostics Inc, Princeton, NJ) through the needle – tip in the intervertebral foramen is inferior to the pedicle – bupivacaine (2–3 ml) and a different steroid are injected. As mentioned earlier, there have been case reports of inadvertent strokes that have occurred after cervical nerve blocks performed using particulate steroid (e.g., methylprednisolone acetate). The authors always use a steroid in liquid form (e.g., dexamethasone 12.5 mg).

After injection, the needle is removed, and a small sterile dressing is applied. Again, in addition to pain relief, temporary numbness or muscle weakness may occur.

Sacral Nerve Block

The technique is similar to that for lumbar nerve blocks. When using fluoroscopy, the C-arm is steeply angulated toward the patient's head. The sacral foramina are ultimately

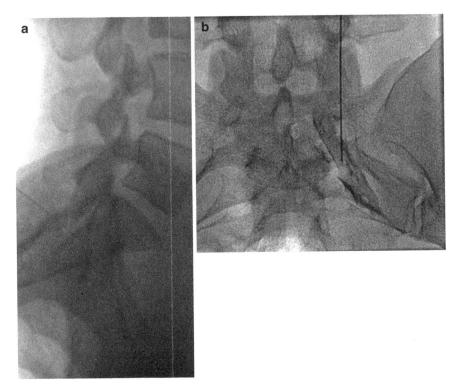

Fig. 6.3 (**a, b**) Sacral nerve block

projected as symmetric ovals. The appropriate level is prepped and draped, skin and tissues anesthetized, and a 22 gauge needle is advanced. On the lateral projection, the needle tip is advanced until the tip is halfway through the thickness of the sacral vertebral body. The technique (i.e., contrast injection), dose of steroid, and volume of bupivacaine injected is generally the same as for lumbar nerve blocks. See Fig. 6.3a, b.

Epidural Spine Injection

Epidural spine injection may prove useful in patients with multilevel spine disease (i.e., spinal stenosis, severe multilevel disc bulges, and degenerative bone disease resulting in spinal canal narrowing, etc.). The technique is similar to myelography except the thecal sac is not punctured (i.e., no CSF is obtained).

After informed consent, the patient is placed prone. The lower back is generally the most common anatomic site chosen. A towel or blanket roll placed across the abdomen may temporarily increase lumbar kyphosis and assist in entering the epidural space (i.e., the patient lays on a rolled up towel or blanket during the procedure). The site is prepped and draped, and local anesthetic is injected in the skin and subcutaneous tissues. A 22 gauge spinal needle is advanced under biplane fluoroscopic guidance. The needle may be advanced

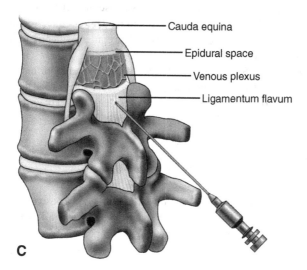

Cauda equina

Epidural space

Venous plexus

Ligamentum flavum

C

Fig. 6.4 Epidural injection

between the spinous processes or a paramedian (parasagittal) approach may be used. See Figs. 6.1b and 6.4. The latter is useful when there is heavy interspinous ligament calcification. Careful, slow needle advancements are required so as not to puncture the dura. Should one enter the thecal sac and obtain CSF, the needle tip must be withdrawn and the tip repositioned. It is theoretically best to choose a different spinal level so as to avoid inadvertent injection of bupivacaine/steroid into the thecal sac, the latter resulting in spinal anesthesia.

To determine if the epidural space has been entered, the needle stylet is removed and the operator watches for CSF. If no CSF is found, a small amount of Isovue-M®200 (Bracco Diagnostics Inc, Princeton, NJ) iodinated contrast is injected. One should see amorphous-shaped contrast spreading in the epidural space. The contrast is at the margins of the neural canal and on the lateral view does not have the characteristic dependent layering as one sees during myelography. On the AP view, the contrast generally spreads out and no nerve roots are outlined.

Once confirmed to be in the epidural space, the authors inject bupivacaine (generally 5 ml of preservative free 0.25% or 0.5%) plus the steroid (generally 80 mg of methylprednisolone acetate). The needle is removed, and a sterile dressing is applied. The patient's head is elevated to theoretically allow the medications injected into the epidural space to slowly move caudally.

Hints, Technical Pitfalls, and Pearls

For pain management, the anesthetic is mixed with the steroid. For thoracic or lumbar nerve blocks, methylprednisolone acetate (Depo-Medrol®, Pfizer Inc, New York, NY) is used. This milky white drug "settles out" in the syringe. It is microparticulate and therefore should not be used for cervical blocks. Use of particulate steroids has rarely been associated with strokes, presumably due to inadvertent injection into a vessel. For cervical blocks, dexamethasone liquid is used. For epidural injections, methylprednisolone acetate may be used.

Needle choice may be operator preference, but some authors have demonstrated a decreased incidence of spinal fluid leak and subsequent spinal headache with the use of smaller needles [8, 9]. However, fine gauge needles that are 29G or smaller are technically more difficult to use and may lead to procedure failure.

Postoperative Care, Discharge Instructions, and Follow-up

Some patients may have conscious sedation and should go to a postanesthesia care unit for adequate recovery. Most patients are not sedated and awake following the procedure. However, each patient may also need to stay for a short period of 1–4 h simply for observation. As spinal injections are relatively low risk, most patients may be discharged home the same day.

Follow-up cross-sectional imaging is not necessary. A follow-up clinic visit for the patient at 4–6 weeks post procedure is helpful to assess pain relief, review the effectiveness and/or durability of recent treatment, and to decide if further injections are necessary. Patients that have received steroids should be questioned regarding their experience with associated side effects.

Outcomes

Systematic reviews have provided strong evidence that nerve blocks and epidural injections have been effective in providing pain relief to patients with lower back pain. More moderate evidence has shown these procedures to be effective in relieving pain from the thoracic area. In addition, nerve blocks have been shown to be especially accurate in diagnosing lumbar and cervical facet join pain [10].

Epidural steroid injections have shown strong evidence of pain relief for lumbar radicular pain in the short-term period of less than 6 weeks. However, long-term pain relief greater than 6 weeks has been moderate to limited. On the other hand, epidural injections for cervical radicular pain provided moderate evidence of pain relief [11].

Complications

Some patients will experience specific neurologic sequelae after nerve root injection including increased spinal pain, non-positional headache, or vasovagal reactions [12]. Steroid effects can include fluid retention, increased glucose levels mood swings, skin changes, and pain flare [12]. Steroid side effects are more likely to occur in patients given high-dose steroids over a short treatment interval.

Complications with any of these injection procedures are rare, but they do exist. They include infection, bleeding into the epidural space with possible spinal cord compression, inadvertent injection of steroid into a blood vessel or the thecal sac (resulting in spinal anesthesia), and spinal headache due to cerebrospinal fluid leak.

The incidence of spinal headache following epidural injection is approximately 2–12% with a 26G needle [9]. Most cases of leak resolve without further intervention. If spinal fluid leak persists, then a blood patch may need to be applied [13].

Rare cases of stroke have been reported during cervical nerve block, either due to inadvertent intravascular injection of air or particulate steroids, or possibly vasospasm even at a distance from the site of injection [14]. Vascular damage has been reported with devastating sequelae following cervical spine transforaminal nerve root block [15].

Summary and Conclusions

Spinal pain management is considered a unique discipline all to itself. Etiologies are multifactorial, and usually a multidisciplinary approach is required in order to achieve treatment success. The Interventional Radiologist can play a pivotal role, providing epidural and spinal injections for diagnostic and therapeutic ends. Evidence supports the use of these methods for accurate diagnosis of lumbar radicular spinal and facet joint pain as well as for all radicular pain relief in the short term. While long-term pain relief is usually not possible, these techniques may also continue to be very important for symptomatic patients as a bridge to more definitive therapy in the spine.

References

1. Pitts SR, Niska RW, Xu J, Burt CW. National Hospital Ambulatory Medical Care Survey: 2006 emergency department summary. National health statistics reports; no 7. Hyattsville, MD: National Center for Health Statistics. 2008.
2. Leboeuf-Yde C, Nielsen J, Kyvik KO, Fejer R, Hartvigsen J. Pain in the lumbar, thoracic or cervical regions: do age and gender matter? A population based study of 34,902 Danish twins 20–71 years of age. BMC Musculoskel Disord. 2009;10:39.
3. Dunn KM. Extending conceptual frameworks: life course epidemiology for the study of back pain. BMC Musculoskelet Disord. 2010;11:23.
4. Eckel TS, Bartynski WS. Epidural steroid injections and selective nerve root blocks. Tech Vasc Interv Radiol. 2009;12(1):11–21.
5. Link SC, el-Khoury GY, Guilford WB. Percutaneous epidural and nerve root block and percutaneous lumbar sympatholysis. Radiol Clin North Am. 1998;36(3):509–21.
6. Waldman SD. Lumbar epidural nerve block. Interventional pain management. 2nd ed. Philadelphia: WB Saunders; 2000. p. 324–439.
7. Strub WM, Brown TA, Ying J, Hoffmann M, Ernst RJ, Bulas RV. Translaminar cervical epidural steroid injection: short-term results and factors influencing outcome. J Vasc Interv Radiol. 2007;18(9):1151–5.
8. Flaatten H, Rodt S, Rosland J, Vamnes J. Postoperative headache in young patients after spinal anaesthesia. Anaesthesia. 1987;42:202–5.

9. Flaatten H, Rodt SA, Vamnes J, Rosland J, Wisborg T, Koller ME. Postdural puncture headache. A comparison between 26 and 29 gauge needles in young patients. Anaesthesia. 1989;44:147–9.

10. Boswell MV, Shah RV, Everett CR, Sehgal N, McKenzie Brown AM, Abdi S, et al. Interventional techniques in the management of chronic spinal pain: evidence-based practice guidelines. Pain Physician. 2005;8(1):1–47.

11. Abdi S, Luca LF. Role of epidural steroids in the management of chronic spinal pain: a systematic review of effectiveness and complications. Pain Physician. 2005;8(1):127–43.

12. Botwin KP, Castellanos R, Rao S, et al. Complications of fluoroscopically guided interlaminar cervical epidural injections. Arch Phys Med Rehabil. 2003;84:627–33.

13. Turnbull DK, Shepherd DB. Postdural puncture headache: pathogenesis, prevention and treatment. Br J Anaesth. 2003;91(5):718–29.

14. Ziai WC, Ardelt AA, Llinas RH. Brainstem stroke following uncomplicated cervical epidural steroid injection. Arch Neurol. 2006;63:1643–6.

15. Rozin L, Rozin R, Koehler SA, et al. Death during transforaminal epidural steroid nerve root block (C7) due to perforation of the left vertebral artery. Am J Forensic Med Pathol. 2003;24:351–5.

Part IV

Lower Extremity Venous Interventions

Lower Extremity Venous Ablation and Sclerotherapy

7

Albert K. Chun, Aaron Himchak, Jason B. Katzen, Chad Baarson, Anthony C. Venbrux, and Nadia J. Khati

Introduction

Venous insufficiency of the lower extremities is common and may present with clinical severity ranging from asymptomatic spider veins to painful varicose veins accompanied by edema and tissue loss. Varicose veins occur in up to 23% of men and 39% of women [1].

Surgical ligation (or stripping) of incompetent superficial veins was once the only option for definitive treatment of symptomatic venous insufficiency. Minimally invasive alternatives, such as endovenous thermal ablation, have become popular over the last decade as these techniques offer effective treatment and fast recovery.

Pathophysiology

Venous blood flow in the lower extremity is primarily affected by muscular contraction and the presence of functional valves. Muscular contraction compresses the deep veins of the lower extremity and forces valves open in one direction (cephalad). Blood traveling in the opposite direction, as with gravity or with a Valsalva maneuver, forces these valves to close. When these valves fail, bidirectional flow occurs, and increased retrograde hydrostatic pressure may be transmitted from the deep veins to superficial veins. Small superficial veins enlarge and may become cosmetic blemishes known as telangiectasias. Larger superficial veins become elongated and tortuous, resulting in varicose veins [2]. Increased venous pressure also impairs tissue oxygenation (by reducing capillary inflow) and may result in edema of the surrounding tissue.

The etiology of venous incompetence is multifactorial and may include increased intra-abdominal pressure from obesity or chronic constipation, increased hydrostatic

A.K. Chun (✉)
Department of Radiology, Division of Interventional Radiology,
The George Washington University Medical Center, Washington, DC, USA
e-mail: achun@mfa.gwu.edu

E.A. Ignacio and A.C. Venbrux (eds.), *Women's Health in Interventional Radiology*,
DOI 10.1007/978-1-4419-5876-1_7, © Springer Science+Business Media, LLC 2012

venous pressure from prolonged standing, venous thrombosis, and familial traits [3]. Female hormonal influences have been suggested as a possible etiology for venous incompetence as most varicose veins that arise in pregnancy do so in the first trimester. The small size of the gravid uterus at this point would exclude a mass effect, increase in blood flow, or iliac venous occlusion as a cause of venous incompetence [4].

Clinical Manifestations

Varicose veins are a prevalent condition. They are found in 10.4–23.0% of men and 29.5–39.0% of women [4]. The clinical sequela of varicose veins goes beyond cosmetics, as some patients initially experience aching pain, fatigue, or night cramps [5]. These symptoms are usually worse with prolonged standing, during a woman's premenstrual period, or in warm weather. Often, the cause of these symptoms is unrecognized by both patients and physicians.

If untreated, approximately half of patients with significant superficial venous insufficiency will develop symptoms of chronic venous insufficiency, including lower extremity edema, eczema, pigmentation, hemorrhage, and ulceration of the skin [5]. Patients may develop corona phlebectasia, a condition with findings of multiple small blue reticular ("spider") veins that crown the proximal ankle. Long-standing venous disease can cause atrophie blanche (ivory white, smooth scar tissue, often within a hyperpigmented areola), lipodermatosclerosis (scarring of the skin and fat with associated discoloration and pain), or ulceration of the skin.

Physicians should attempt intervention to reduce/relieve symptoms as well as to prevent disease progression.

The clinical status, etiology, anatomy, and pathophysiology (CEAP) classification takes into account many factors including the severity, cause, anatomic site, and specific abnormality of patients with venous disease of the lower extremity [6]. The elements and levels of this classification system are defined next. The use of a classification system such as this improves the communication between physicians of different specialties:

Class	Description
C0	No visible or palpable signs of venous disease
C1	Telangiectasias or reticular veins
C2	Varicose veins, distinguished from reticular veins by a diameter ≥3 mm
C3	Edema
C4	Changes in skin and subcutaneous tissue
C4a	Eczema, pigmentation (and additionally corona phlebectasia)
C4b	Lipodermatosclerosis or atrophie blanche
C5	Healed venous ulcer
C6	Active venous ulcer

Several other classification systems exist including the Venous Disability Score (VDS), the Venous Clinical Severity Score (VCSS), and the Venous Segmental Disease Score (VSDS). The Venous Severity Score (VSS) is a summation of these systematic scores. Formal classification of a patient's venous disease will support uniform understanding as well as promote consistent treatment for these patients.

Anatomy

Lower Extremity Venous Anatomy

The veins of the lower extremity are divided into the deep and superficial venous systems. The superficial veins of the lower extremity include the *great (or greater or long) saphenous vein* (GSV) and the *small (or short or lesser) saphenous vein* (SSV). See Fig. 7.1a, b. The great saphenous vein originates in the medial dorsal portion of the foot and extends into the femoral vein, just inferior to the inguinal ligament (*saphenofemoral junction*). The small saphenous vein originates in the lateral foot and extends toward the knee, where it joins the popliteal vein (*saphenopopliteal junction*). The superficial venous drainage of the lateral aspect of the lower extremity is termed the lateral venous complex. The lateral venous complex drains into the anterolateral thigh vein, which joins the saphenofemoral junction.

There are several sites where the deep and the superficial veins connect. In addition to the saphenofemoral and saphenopopliteal junctions, four major perforating veins pierce the muscular fascia and connect the deep and superficial systems. In the proximal and distal thigh, these veins are named *Hunter and Dodd perforating veins*, respectively. Paratibial perforating veins in the calf are referred to as *Boyd perforators* and posterior tibial perforators, near the ankle, are called *Cockett perforators*. The *vein of Giacomini* is a superficial vein that connects the great saphenous and short saphenous veins at the posteromedial aspect of the lower extremity. These communications are important anatomic landmarks and represent the chief pathways for the development of superficial varicosities.

Imaging

Duplex ultrasound is the dominant modality used for preprocedure and postprocedure evaluation. Like many IR procedures, the scanning physician may also be the future operator, and this linear relationship with the patient will help provide for the best outcomes and patient satisfaction. If the operator was not able to personally scan the patient at the previous visit, a complete review of the images and details of flow dynamics should be carefully reviewed prior to the endovenous therapy of choice.

The deep venous system must always be evaluated to exclude the presence of deep vein thrombosis (DVT). The deep venous system should also be assessed for reflux prior to

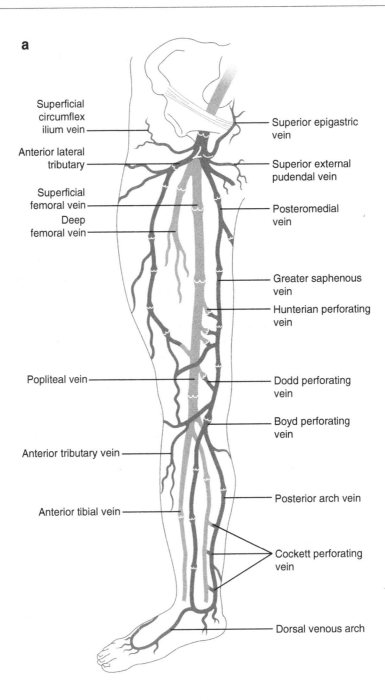

a

Superficial circumflex ilium vein

Anterior lateral tributary

Superficial femoral vein

Deep femoral vein

Popliteal vein

Anterior tributary vein

Anterior tibial vein

Superior epigastric vein

Superior external pudendal vein

Posteromedial vein

Greater saphenous vein

Hunterian perforating vein

Dodd perforating vein

Boyd perforating vein

Posterior arch vein

Cockett perforating vein

Dorsal venous arch

Fig. 7.1 (**a, b**) Venous anatomy of the lower extremity

b

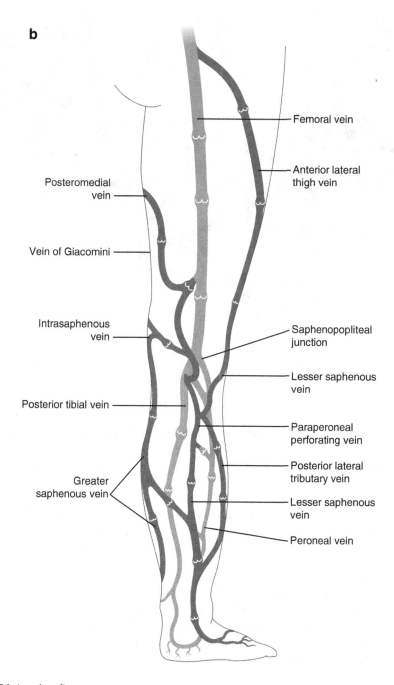

Fig. 7.1 (continued)

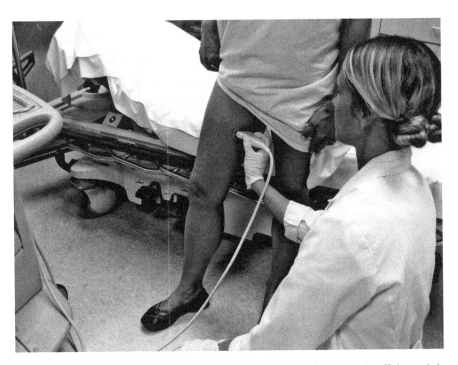

Fig. 7.2 Photograph of patient during ultrasound. When searching for venous insufficiency, it is best to scan the patient standing. The patient may lean slightly on a high stool or examination table for extra support

superficial vein closure. If clinically indicated, deep venous insufficiency may be further evaluated with a digital subtraction venogram. Once patency and competence of the deep venous system have been established, the superficial venous system is sonographically evaluated.

The search for DVT may be done with the patient supine, but the evaluation for superficial venous insufficiency is best performed with the patient standing. The patient's weight is supported by the contralateral (unscanned) lower extremity. The patient may lean slightly on a high stool or examination table for extra support during the examination. See Fig. 7.2.

First, one should acquire axial and longitudinal images in grayscale of the entire superficial venous system from the GSV through the SFJ to the SSV and the lowest varicosities. See Figs. 7.3a–d and 7.4a–d. When a vein is insufficient, there will be dilatation, and diameter measurements should be recorded. The insufficient vein will usually be dilated below a high pressure leak. The diameter may then decrease as the flow is decompressed to another refluxing tributary or to a competent perforator draining to the deep venous system.

One then checks for reflux by instructing the patient to Valsalva or by manual augmentation of the vein (by squeezing the thigh or calf). Color and power Doppler imaging are helpful to identify the reflux, but may underestimate the degree of abnormal flow. Pulsed wave Doppler is best for identifying and quantifying venous reflux, as it is more sensitive and specific [7]. It should be noted that, in normal veins with normal valvular function, there will be a small amount of retrograde flow before valve closure. Under dynamic exam, the presence of significant reflux is characterized by retrograde flow after releasing the distal compression placed below the scanned segment. A duration (or time to valve closure) greater than 0.5 s is the minimum criteria to define reflux. If reflux is noted, the

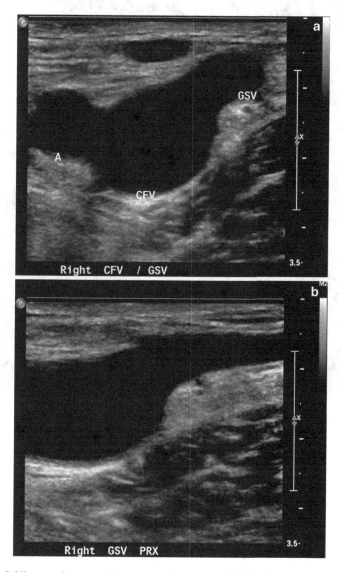

Fig. 7.3 (a–d) Ultrasound images of the great saphenous vein (GSV). Note the relationship to the common femoral vein (CFV)

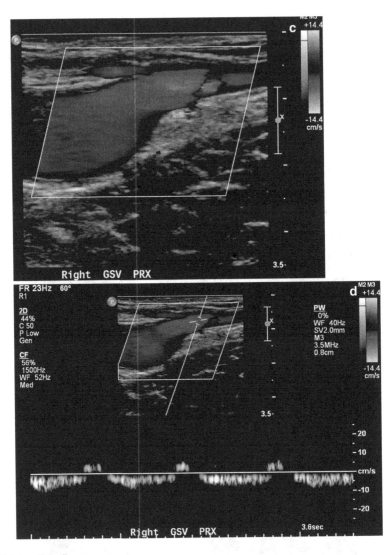

Fig. 7.3 (continued)

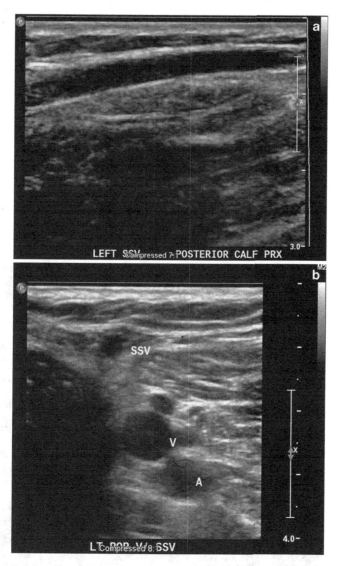

Fig. 7.4 (**a–d**) Ultrasound images of the small saphenous vein (SSV). Note the relationship to the popliteal vein

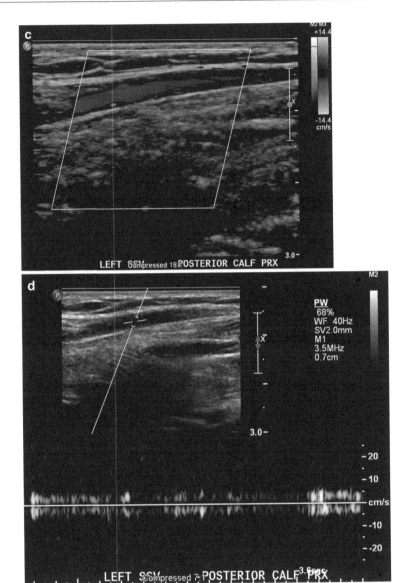

Fig. 7.4 (continued)

location (saphenofemoral or saphenopopliteal junction, proximal/distal GSV or SSV) and duration of reflux should be documented.

Any branching veins arising from the GSV or SSV should be noted, as well as the presence of thrombus.

During or immediately after the scan, it is helpful to complete a venous map for accurate documentation. Examples of common patterns of varicose veins are shown in Fig. 7.5a–d.

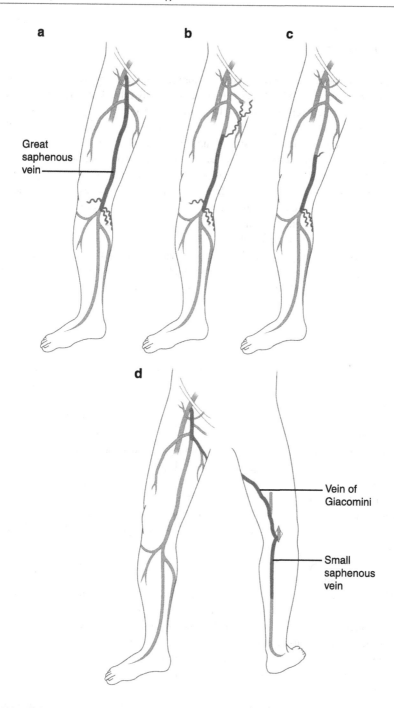

Fig. 7.5 (a–d) Common patterns of varicose veins

Patient Encounter

Many patients who seek some type of therapy for their venous problems may desire either a cosmetic improvement in their lower extremities or simply relief from the typical pain and other sequelae of their venous disease. These two groups are not mutually exclusive, however, as many patients who have serious symptomatic venous disease also desire aesthetic benefit. Conversely, evaluation of patient candidates who are concerned with the superficial appearance of their legs may reveal significant underlying venous insufficiency.

Physicians and their patients have many choices in terms of therapy, and surgery versus endoluminal therapy is a primary branch point of the decision-making tree. Endoluminal options are appealing because of significantly reduced perioperative morbidity [5]. Many vein centers offer endovenous treatments primarily, and then move to surgical options only if the noninvasive methods have failed.

A clinic visit including history, physical examination, and a full review of the treatment options is absolutely essential in order to set realistic patient expectations and achieve overall success for the patient.

Indications and Contraindications

Conservative measures initially include use of compression stockings and elevation of the legs. Should this fail, endovenous treatment options may be considered. Sclerotherapy is a procedure in which medication is injected into the vein, leading to occlusion. Endovenous thermal ablation (EVTA) is a procedure in which energy is applied to the vein wall via a catheter, causing occlusion and fibrosis of the treated venous segment.

Sclerotherapy is the current treatment of choice for spider and reticular veins as well as telangiectasias, and this is its singular indication [2].

For symptomatic patients with CEAP class C2 or higher disease, the Multi-Society Consensus Quality Improvement Guidelines do recommend treatment of the venous insufficiency with thermal ablation either via radiofrequency or laser. These treatments are definitely indicated to improve the patient's quality of life [6]. More specifically, radiofrequency ablation is currently indicated for use in closing portions of the incompetent great and lesser saphenous veins, major tributaries of the saphenous veins, perforating veins, and recurrent varicosities after surgery [8].

Thus, reasonable candidates for endovenous therapy will have symptoms including leg pain, heaviness, fatigue, or itching. Other indications include clinical signs of superficial thrombophlebitis, external bleeding, ankle hyperpigmentation, lipodermatosclerosis, atrophie blanche, and venous ulcers [3].

Contraindications to venous endoluminal therapies have not been completely defined. Contraindications may be based on the patient's anatomy as well as on the patient's clinical status.

EVLT and RFA have similar indications and contraindications. Contraindications include obstruction of the deep venous system, sciatic vein reflux, the presence of thrombus in the vessel being treated or a vessel smaller than 2 mm in the supine position [8].

Tortuous veins are a relative contraindication because of the difficulty in passing a catheter through the vessel [8].

Pregnancy/nursing, liver dysfunction, local anesthetic allergy, active infection, an uncorrectable coagulopathy, or hypercoagulable state are all contraindications as defined by the patient's clinical status. Some authors specifically stress the need for caution when using these procedures in thrombophilic patients [2].

The liver is the site of metabolism for anesthetic agents typically used in thermal ablation therapies for venous disease. In patients with liver dysfunction, anesthetic toxicity may result. Specific modifications or alternatives are present for these patients. (See the section on Hints, Technical Pitfalls, and Pearls in this chapter.)

All procedures are done with percutaneous image-guided needle access, and caution is advised to perform endovenous procedures on patients with specific preexisting skin disorders such as Ehler Danlos or other connective tissue disorders, as well as patients with a history of keloid formation. Certainly, cosmesis is not always the primary goal, but patients will want to know what outcomes may be reasonably expected in these settings.

The presence of either a pacemaker or a nerve stimulator is a relative contraindication to venous thermal ablation with radiofrequency.

Compression bandages and/or stockings are uniformly necessary for postoperative care following endovenous treatment. The strong elastic in compression stockings squeezes the calf and thigh muscles and reduces the passive venous refilling that could lead to recanalization after treatment. If a patient cannot wear these for whatever reason, that is a relative contraindication to endovenous therapy. This includes patients with peripheral arterial disease, patients with skin hypersensitivity to compression materials, and patients with any physical/neurologic limitation to wearing compression bandages or stockings.

Patients are encouraged to ambulate soon after the venous interventions, as this will decrease the possible risk for thrombosis in deep veins. For this reason, inability to ambulate adequately is a relative contraindication for endovenous treatment.

Consult and Consent

A full history and physical should be obtained prior to the endovenous procedure. In particular, symptoms of venous insufficiency (leg pain, edema, pruritus, etc.) should be elicited as well as frequency and duration of these symptoms and modifying factors. Patients with venous insufficiency commonly report worsening of symptoms while upright, with activity, and in the evening. Conversely, these symptoms are often decreased while supine, at rest, and in the morning.

It is also important to obtain any history of prior treatment for venous insufficiency such as use of compression stockings, vein stripping, phlebectomy, sclerotherapy, or endovenous ablation.

In women, plans for future pregnancy should be discussed. Symptoms of venous insufficiency are often significantly worse during and after pregnancy, an effect which is thought to be related to increased progesterone levels.

Physical exam and ultrasound examination may be performed at the time of the initial consultation. These both should be performed with the patient standing. Particular attention should be paid to the pattern of venous insufficiency (GSV and/or SSV distribution). Baseline photographic imaging of affected areas is often useful for monitoring treatment progress.

As stated previously, it is extremely important that various treatment options be discussed in full with the patient. A review of the benefits and risks of the various options as discussed next is critical for patient education, clinical success, and ultimate patient satisfaction.

Review of Benefits and Risks of Various Procedures

Sclerotherapy

A significant advantage of foam sclerotherapy is that it is relatively inexpensive as compared to other endovascular techniques. Postprocedure pain is minimal. Another significant advantage of this procedure over surgery is that it can be performed in an outpatient setting and it requires minimal or no anesthesia. This is an important consideration in patients who are poor surgical candidates.

The main limitation to sclerotherapy is that it has been shown to be less effective in the long- term treatment of varicose veins as compared to surgical methods [9]. As a result, consecutive treatment sessions may be necessary to treat a patient with varicose veins. Patients should be informed that sclerotherapy may not be just one procedure but may involve a few procedures as part of an overall process.

Other disadvantages include injecting the vein percutaneously, requiring several needle punctures until desired symptomatic relief and cosmetic effects are achieved. There is also a risk of injecting into an artery. These two drawbacks are diminished when the foam sclerosant is delivered via a catheter [2].

Post-sclerotherapy pigmentation may occur, but there are methods available to treat this. (See Technique section in this chapter.) Serious adverse events are very unusual to rare for this procedure, and include sclerotherapy-induced extravasation necrosis. (See Complications section in this chapter.)

Radiofrequency Ablation

Radiofrequency ablation (RFA) is a minimally invasive technique that can be performed with tumescent local anesthesia or intravenous conscious sedation. In this procedure, a bipolar catheter is placed via fluoroscopic guidance into the lumen of a vessel to deliver a high-frequency alternating current. This causes ionic agitation and local heating, resulting in spasm of the vein. The procedure also permanently denatures the collagen within the vessel wall. The end benefit is destruction of the intima leading to a fibrotic seal within the lumen with a minimal amount of thrombus formation [2].

The Endovenous Obliteration versus Ligation and Vein Stripping (EVOLVeS) trial found other benefits of RFA when compared to surgery. These included faster recovery time and less postoperative pain. Patients were also able to return to work and normal activity sooner. On average, 80% of the RFA group could resume normal activity in a day in comparison to 46% of the surgical group. The average work leave was 4.7 days in the RFA group. Other benefits included earlier cosmetic results, fewer incisions, fewer hematomas, and fewer ecchymoses. In general, the average patient's quality of life improved sooner with RFA treatment as compared to surgery [10, 11].

One significant disadvantage of RFA is cost. RFA is currently the most expensive method to treat varicose veins. The main cost is in the disposable tips used in the devices. Cost-benefit analyses have yet to be undertaken [3]. Body mass index (BMI) is a significant cause for anatomic failure [8].

Even though it is a minimally invasive procedure, RFA is not without risks. The two major adverse events described in the literature are the formation of a deep vein thrombosis (DVT) and a resulting pulmonary embolus. (See Complications section in this chapter.) A review of published case reports indicates the rate of these events to be 1% and 0.3%, respectively [4]. Due to the risk of developing thrombus, early duplex scanning should be considered in patients greater than 50 years of age [12]. Some authors believe that DVT is due to initiating the venous ablation too close to the saphenofemoral junction. Thus, these events might be avoided by modification of technique [2]. Other less serious events can occur from the internal heating of the involved blood vessel. These include paresthesia of the overlying skin (13% median incidence), burns of the overlying skin and soft tissue (2.8% median incidence), clinical thrombophlebitis (3.4% median incidence), and postoperative pain (5% median incidence) [4]. The risk of these events, especially paresthesia and skin burns, can be improved with the use of tumescent anesthesia and great operator experience [2].

Endovenous Laser Therapy

Treatment of varicose veins through endovenous laser therapy (EVLT) is a relatively new treatment option since Boné first reported it in 1999. It was approved for the treatment of varicose veins by the United States Food and Drug Administration (FDA) in January 2002 [2]. This procedure uses a laser with a short wavelength that is delivered via an endovenous laser fiber that is generally 600 μm in diameter. The laser energy locally boils the blood and generates steam bubbles, which then cause a heat injury to the endothelial wall of the vein. The short wavelength used in this procedure has a great tendency to act directly on blood instead of surrounding tissue. This theoretically allows for a high selection of endothelial targets via heat therapy with a lower rate of affecting surrounding tissues [2].

The benefits of EVLT are similar to those of RFA. This technique allows for very specific targeting of vessels through an endoluminal technique without the need for general anesthesia. It avoids the perioperative morbidity of surgery [5]. Because the laser is specific for generating heat within the walls of a varicose vein, it has a lower incidence of damaging surrounding tissue and is less likely to cause a scar [13] It is also less expensive to perform than RFA [8].

Aside from the fact that EVLT is more expensive than sclerotherapy or surgical options, there are few disadvantages to EVLT. There have been few adverse events reported and a low incidence of deep vein thrombosis and pulmonary embolus. Similar to RFA, early duplex scanning should be considered in patients greater than 50 years of age due to the risk of developing thrombus [12]. Studies report ecchymosis and induration to be the most common side effects, with ranges of 23.0–100% and 34.1–100%, respectively [1].

A comparison study of EVLT to surgery performed in 2007 showed that there was no difference in short-term benefits of EVLT in comparison to surgery. It showed that patients returned to work and normal activity at the same rate with a higher cost for EVLT [14]. As this is a newer technique, further investigation is necessary in order to adequately assess the efficacy, benefits, and drawbacks of EVLT.

Bilateral Procedures

Many patients have bilateral venous disease. It would seem reasonable to consider bilateral procedures for these patients in the same day. This is especially true if there is clinical evidence of advanced stages of venous insufficiency, including ulceration and tissue loss, as well as an urgent need for definitive treatment. Additionally, many patients may request bilateral same-day procedures depending on factors such as limited medical leave from work. However, bilateral procedures do carry a theoretical doubled increased risk compared to that of the unilateral procedure for entities such as deep venous thrombosis. Further, compliance with postoperative requirements such as compression stockings and adequate ambulation may present more of a challenge for patients who have had both lower extremities treated.

Patient Preparation

Aside from imaging with venous mapping, no other studies are required.

Some physicians will have baseline protime and prothrombin time drawn on the day of the procedure.

Since compression stockings are needed postoperatively, patients are sized and fitted for them earlier. Usually, these are Class 2 (30–40 mmHg) compression stockings. The patient will bring these stockings to the vein center on the day of the procedure.

The patient does not need to be n.p.o. Patients are instructed to take their morning medications and have a light breakfast. Any oral anticoagulants should be held for at least 1 week prior to the procedure.

Technique

Equipment and Materials

A linear array ultrasound probe with color Doppler should be available for pre- and post-procedure evaluation as well as intraprocedural guidance.

Sclerotherapy Materials

Most operators will need a small needle (23, 25, or 30 gauge) ½ inches long, plastic tubing, and 10–20 ml syringes.

A vein light may be helpful for visualization of smaller veins.

There are several categories of sclerosing agents available. These include osmotic agents, detergents, and alcohol-based agents. These cause vascular injury by altering the surface tension of endothelial cells or by injuring endothelial cells via heavy metal cauterizing effect. Osmotic agents include hypertonic saline and Sclerodex® (Omega Laboratories Ltd, Montreal, Quebec, Canada), a mixture of hypertonic saline and dextrose. Detergent agents include sodium morrhuate (Scleromate®, Glenwood LLC, Englewood, NJ), sodium tetradecyl sulfate (Sotradecol®, AngioDynamics, Latham, NY), and polidocanol (Aethoxysklerol®, Bioform Medical/Merz, Greensboro, NC). Alcohol-based sclerosing agents include glycerin-based agents such as Chromex® (Omega Laboratories Ltd, Montreal, Quebec, Canada).

RFA and Laser Materials

A number of devices are available for endovenous laser or radiofrequency venous ablation. The devices consist of a power source and single-use endovenous ablation catheters. For radiofrequency ablation, an example is the VNUS® Closure system (VNUS Medical Technologies, Covidien, Mansfield, MA). For endovenous laser therapy, an example is the Venacure® System (AngioDynamics, Latham, NY). See Fig. 7.6A-D.

Some operators use a tumescent anesthesia pump that may allow for faster infusion. With the use of a pump and its reservoir, there is no need to refill the anesthesia syringe, and so less needle punctures may be required.

Other tools typically used for these endovenous procedures may include an access needle such as a 19 gauge single wall needle, or a 4 or 5 Fr micropuncture sheath set, as well as a 6 or 7 Fr vascular sheath, and a 0.025 or 0.035 guide wire.

Procedure Start

No local anesthesia is necessary for sclerotherapy, as the discomfort from injectable anesthesia may be greater than discomfort from the injections of the sclerotherapy procedure alone. Additionally, access into small veins may be obscured by injectable anesthetics. Some operators may elect to apply a topical anesthetic prior to the procedure, although the application of creams over the treatment areas may increase the risk of infection or inflammation, particularly while the compression stocking is in place.

For endovenous thermal ablation, local anesthesia with lidocaine is typically used at the access site, in addition to tumescent anesthesia. No other anesthesia is required, and this allows patients to eat before the procedure and leave the facility immediately after the procedure. Some centers may offer an oral sedative or anxiolytic such as lorazepam immediately before the procedure in addition to local anesthesia. Intravenous conscious sedation may also be offered. While allowing for a great degree of pain control and amnesia, the use of intravenous conscious sedation introduces several requirements. These patients must be n.p.o. prior to the procedure and must be accompanied to and from the procedure by an adult. The patient's full history and physical examination should be reviewed, with particular attention to a history of sleep apnea, cardiopulmonary disease, or any other anesthesia risk factors.

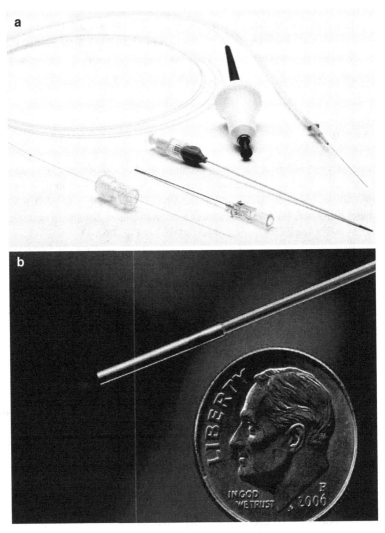

Fig. 7.6 (a) The VenaCure EVLT® PVAK procedure kit. (b) NeverTouch® gold tip laser fiber. (c) Delta diode laser unit. (d) Tumescent delivery system anesthesia pump (AngioDynamics, Latham, NY) (Courtesy of AngioDynamics, Inc. With permission)

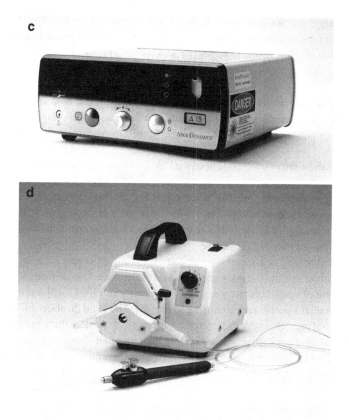

Fig. 7.6 (continued)

The patient is placed on the procedure table with the treatment areas exposed. For sclerotherapy, the treatment areas may simply be swabbed with alcohol prior to treatment. Generally, the patient is placed supine for access to the great saphenous vein and prone for access to the short saphenous vein. The lower extremity is prepared in sterile fashion and draped for endovenous thermal ablation procedures.

Step by Step

Sclerotherapy

Because sclerotherapy involves injecting a liquid or foam solution into a vessel, vessels too small to cannulate can be targeted with this treatment. It is ideal for vessels smaller than 4 mm in diameter [3]. For larger veins, such as perforating veins, the target vein is accessed using ultrasound guidance and a micropuncture set. Care should be taken to note junctions of perforating veins with deep veins, as injection of the sclerosant into the deep system increases the risk of DVT.

Severe allergic reactions have been reported in the use of sodium tetradecyl sulfate, and so manufacturer recommendations advise a test injection of 0.5 ml into the varicosity with a waiting period of a few hours. Emergency resuscitation equipment should be accessible.

Ultrasound is also used to monitor injection of the sclerosant and thrombosis of the target vein.

For spider and reticular veins, the skin should be cleaned, and the veins are accessed directly using a small needle attached to plastic tubing and a syringe containing the sclerosant. After each puncture, gentle aspiration is performed to confirm needle position within the target vein.

In general, there are two methods described for venous sclerotherapy:

1. Traditional sclerotherapy involves injecting an irritant liquid into a vessel. The liquid injures the endothelium of the vessel with subsequent secondary wall attached local thrombus formation. The veins then undergo fibrous transformation into a fibrous cord. This fibrous cord does not recanalize.
2. Foam sclerotherapy is a specific technique of mixing air or gas such as CO_2 into a syringe with sclerosing agents, creating a foam sclerosant. Use of foam sclerotherapy for treatment of venous disease was described as early as 1939 [3, 15] and may be more efficacious than a pure liquid sclerosing agent [16]. The foam displaces blood from the treated vessel and allows for the sclerosant to contact the endothelium more uniformly, thus increasing the effective surface area of the agent and decreasing the amount and concentration of necessary sclerosing agent. It also prevents the sclerosant from being readily washed out. Foam also causes venospasm, further aiding the closure of the target vessel [3].

Over the years, the foam technique has been adjusted to improve upon safety, efficacy, simplicity, speed, and clinical reproducibility. The primary technical factors that have been investigated are (1) the size of the bubbles, (2) the tensioactive property of the sclerosing agent, and (3) the methods by which the foam is prepared and maintained throughout the procedure. The most important variable appears to be the size of the bubbles. A small bubble size is desired because it ensures a great concentration of sclerosing agent delivered and reduced hemodilution, leading to great sclerosant efficacy.

The sclerosant is always injected slowly until blanching of the target veins is seen. After the injection, the needle is then removed, and gentle manual compression is applied over the injection site. If there is extravasation, the injection should be discontinued. Some operators treat areas of possible extravasation with hyaluronidase 75 units [17].

After sclerotherapy, compression bandages are typically applied over the treated area [3].

RFA and EVLT

For both methods of endovenous thermal ablation (RFA and EVLT), the patient should have the treatment area marked on the skin using ultrasound guidance. Perforating veins, accessory veins, and junctions with deep veins should also be marked immediately before the procedure.

Fig. 7.7 Sagittal ultrasound image of needle access into GSV. Note the anechoic fluid (tumescent anesthesia) surrounding the ablation catheter (intraluminal linear echogenicity)

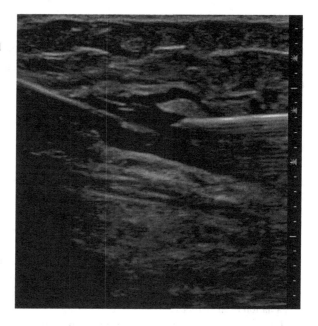

To facilitate venous access, it may be beneficial to tilt the patient in a reverse Trendelenburg position to promote venodilation. Access should be achieved in the lowest incompetent segment. This is commonly done using a micropuncture set with a transitional dilator and ultrasound guidance. The micropuncture sheath is then exchanged over a guidewire for an introducer sheath which is compatible with the ablation device. The wire and dilator are removed, and the RFA or EVLT device may then be advance coaxially through the sheath.

The device tip should be placed approximately 1–2 cm caudal to the saphenofemoral junction for GSV ablations. For SSV ablations, the device tip should be placed caudal to the junction of the SSV and popliteal vein. Device position should be confirmed by ultrasound and (if visible) by transillumination. It is crucial to avoid positioning the device within the deep veins as this may result in ablation of competent veins and/or DVT.

After the device tip is in position, tumescent anesthesia is delivered around the target vein (Fig. 7.7). For tumescent anesthesia, lidocaine is diluted with normal saline to a concentration of 0.10%: 30 ml of lidocaine 1% diluted in 270 ml normal saline solution. If the procedure will be performed on both lower extremities (bilateral) at the same sitting, this concentration may be halved, i.e., the volume of dilutant is doubled. This will limit the total lidocaine dose to <4.5 mg/kg in a standard 70 kg patient [18].

Tumescent anesthesia involves injection of the local anesthetic using ultrasound guidance circumferentially around the target vein. Tumescent anesthesia serves several purposes: (1) external compression and emptying of the target vein, (2) maximization of wall contact between vein wall and the device, (3) creation of a thermal barrier (heat sink) between the device and surrounding anatomic structures, and (4) mild local anesthesia. The thermal barrier may be especially important when the target veins are less than 10 mm from the skin surface.

Once tumescent anesthesia has been delivered along the length of the target segment, the device is activated and withdrawn. For EVLT, the goal is delivery of a minimum of 80 J/cm. For RFA, the target temperature is 85°C with a pullback rate of 2 cm/min.

Hemostasis is achieved at the access site with manual compression. Sterile dressings are applied and the leg is then wrapped and placed in a graduated compression stocking for 7–14 days. The patient may ambulate immediately.

Hints, Technical Pitfalls, and Pearls

If possible, photographic documentation of the affected limb(s) should be obtained before and after the procedure. This may serve as a useful reference for the practitioner and may help manage patient expectations.

For all percutaneous treatment methods, practitioners should strive to obtain access with a single puncture to avoid venospasm. Venospasm may resolve by placing the patient in a reverse Trendelenburg position or by having the patient stand and walk. If spasm does not resolve, treatment may be postponed. Accessing the vein at a higher (more proximal) location is often unsuccessful and is not recommended as the treatment results in suboptimal ablation of the target vein.

If patients have either liver dysfunction or an allergy to the anesthetic agent, one may use saline for tumescent infiltration prior to thermal ablation [19].

Post-sclerotherapy pigmentation occurs in 30% of patients. This hyperpigmentation may be decreased or prevented if the thrombus is removed 1–3 weeks after sclerotherapy. Microthrombectomy has been shown to improve the clinical results for patients with small 1 mm or less size treated veins [20].

Postoperative, Discharge, and Follow-Up

Following the procedure, the patient receiving intravenous conscious sedation must be monitored prior to discharge. Discharge criteria generally include stable vital signs and a return to baseline level of consciousness with appropriate pain control.

The treatment protocol for postoperative pain medication upon discharge varies widely among institutions. While some physicians recommend only acetaminophen and NSAIDS for pain over a 1 week period, others will give the patient a short course of narcotic pain medication. Aspirin-based products should be avoided.

Patients are instructed that all skin incisions and injection sites be kept clean and dry until healed. For sclerotherapy, the injection sites are especially prone to hyperpigmentation. Therefore, patients are counseled to avoid exposure to direct sunlight for 3–4 weeks after each injection.

Although patients are encouraged to ambulate after these endovenous procedures, they are restricted from vigorous exercise for approximately 1 week after the procedure since this may cause the ablated veins to reopen. Some operators also will advise against hot baths.

Different centers will have specific compression stocking regimens. Immediately after the procedure, the leg is wrapped in a stretch compression adhesive bandage such as

Comprilan® (Jobst, Charlotte, NC). Most physicians will have patients keep this in place for the first 72 h. After this interval, patients may wear their fitted compression stockings from waking in the morning to bedtime at night for another 10 days.

Interval follow-up is essential. Some operators prefer to have a follow-up ultrasound in 24 h. An initial follow-up should be scheduled for 10–14 days after each procedure. This visit coincides with completion of the stocking regimen, and signs of clinical improvement may not be initially evident. Complications such as thrombosis or wound infection may be addressed in a timely fashion (e.g., needle aspiration, anticoagulation, or antibiotics). Longer follow-up at 3–6 month intervals allows for more complete assessment of clinical or cosmetic improvement.

Outcomes

Sclerotherapy

The efficacy of foam sclerotherapy is greatly dependent upon the preparation of the foam itself. The two main preparation methods are the Monfreux technique and the Tessari technique. The Monfreux technique generates foam by drawing air into a single syringe with a tightly closed tip that contains the sclerosing agent, thus generating large air bubbles. The Tessari technique uses two syringes, one containing a liquid and the other containing air, and involves mixing the air and liquid through a three-way stopcock between the syringes. This double syringe technique generates smaller bubbles. A 3-year study from Italy has determined the immediate success rate of the Monfreux and Tessari techniques for medium and large veins to be 88.1% and 93.3%, respectively [3]. Of the initial successes, about 80–90% of treated medium to large vessels remain occluded after 3 years [2]. Studies have shown that sclerotherapy has a great initial success than surgery within the first year of treatment. This initial success, however, quickly diminishes with surgery being a more effective treatment at 3 years and at 5 years [21].

RFA

Several trials have been published comparing the efficacy of RFA to traditional surgical and nonsurgical methods of treatment of varicose veins. The Endovenous Obliteration versus Ligation and Vein Stripping (EVOLVeS) trial examined the efficacy of RFA compared to the conventional surgical method of ligation and venous stripping for the treatment of great saphenous vein varicosities. It found that the efficacy of RFA was similar to that of conventional surgical methods at the immediate and 2 year follow-up marks (Fig. 7.8a, b). The great saphenous vein was successfully treated in 95% of the RFA group in comparison to 100% in the surgical group immediately after each procedure. At the 2 year follow-up, the recurrence rate of varicose veins was 14% for the RFA group and 21% for the surgical group [10, 11].

There are several ways in which RFA can fail. The veins could fail to close initially, previously closed veins can recanalize, and the area can become neovascularized. Literature

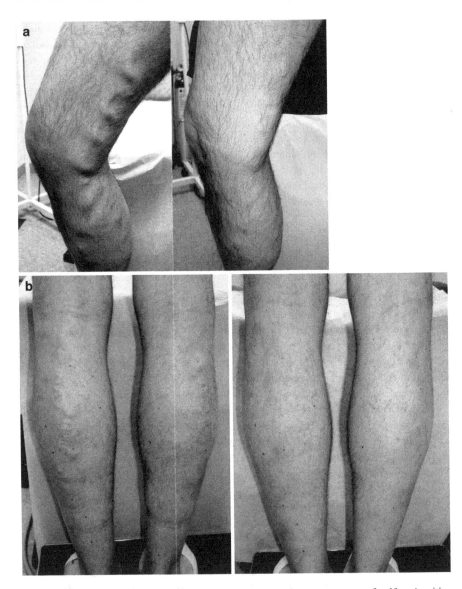

Fig. 7.8 (**a**, **b**) Photographs of patients. Pre- and postprocedure appearance of calf varicosities (Courtesy of AngioDynamics, Inc. With permission)

reviews have found that 0–18.7% of treated varicose veins remain patent initially as compared to a 0–12.5% failure rate with surgery. Long-term failure of the procedure after an initial success by either recanalization of the treated vein or neovascularization has been found to have a median incidence rate of 8% in published literature [1].

EVLT

One of the first clinical trials to examine the efficacy of EVLT was performed in 2001. This trial used a laser with a wavelength of 810 nm to treat a varicose great saphenous vein. At 1 week, 97% of patients had a closed great saphenous vein [5]. At 2 years, there was only a 7% recurrence rate [22]. Because this technique is new, there is no study available comparing EVLT to surgery at long-term follow-up (e.g., 10 years). In other published studies, EVLT proved to have a similar efficacy in comparison to surgery at 6 months.

Complications

Significant adverse reactions for all percutaneous venous interventions are uncommon.

Sclerotherapy of small superficial veins may result in focal erythema or inflammation. Extravasation necrosis may occur with sodium tetradecyl 0.5%. This complication may be decreased with the use of hyaluronidase [17].

Review of the current literature reveals several possible adverse events from endovenous thermal ablation. Thrombophlebitis may occur, which may be relieved by aspiration of thrombus. Other possible complications include nerve damage and allergic reactions to the sclerosing agents. More severe complications are rare but include pulmonary embolism, skin necrosis, problems associated with an intra-arterial injection of the sclerosant, and deep venous thrombosis. Less serious events include cosmetic blemishes over the treated site such as skin thickening, staining, pigmentation, and pain at the injection site [2].

The most common complications from EVLT and RFA include ecchymosis, hematoma, and infection. Deep venous thrombosis (DVT) and pulmonary embolism are feared, but infrequent. The incidence of DVT is 0.3% for laser ablation and 0.4% for RF ablation [6]. Additionally, skin burns, paresthesia, and clinical thrombophlebitis may also occur. Early experience with endovenous therapies showed higher incidence of skin burns near 4%, with subsequently lower values following the introduction and more routine use of tumescent anesthesia [6].

In EVLT, problems with incorrect placement of the laser have also been reported [2]. There was one mortality reported with this procedure; a patient died 6 weeks after EVLT due to a mesenteric infarction. This event was not considered to be a result of the procedure [2]. As with RFA, minor complications of the EVLT procedure include postoperative pain, ecchymosis, induration, bleeding complications, and phlebitis.

Summary and Conclusions

Superficial venous insufficiency is a common problem that may result in significant pain and swelling in the affected limb. Left untreated, this may lead to more severe problems such as thrombophlebitis, thromboembolism, or venous stasis ulcers. Open surgery for

Table 7.1 Summary of indications, advantages, drawbacks, and side effects of endovenous therapies

	Sclerotherapy	Radiofrequency ablation	Endovascular laser therapy
Indication	Primarily for veins <4 mm, spider and reticular veins, and telangiectasias	Ablation of great and lesser saphenous veins	Ablation of great and lesser saphenous veins
Advantages	Inexpensive, can be administered percutaneously	Fast recovery, long-term efficacy comparable to surgery	Less expensive than RFA with similar benefits
Drawbacks	Decreased efficacy in the presence of venous reflux	Increased cost	Increased cost
Side effects	Pulmonary Embolism (PE), necrosis and ulceration of overlying skin, Deep Venous Thrombus (DVT), skin discoloration	DVT, PE, skin burns, paresthesias, ecchymosis thrombophlebitis, pain	DVT, PE, skin burns, paresthesias, ecchymosis thrombophlebitis, pain

venous insufficiency has become widely replaced by percutaneous procedures that may be performed in an outpatient setting. With appropriate patient selection, careful technique, and attentive follow-up, these methods may be used alone or in combination to provide effective treatment with minimal risk to the patient with venous disease.

A summary of endovenous therapies is outlined in Table 7.1.

References

1. Leopardi D et al. Systematic review of treatments for varicose veins. Ann Vasc Surg. 2009;23:264–76.
2. Sadick NS. Advances in the Treatment of Varicose Veins: Ambulatory Phlebectomy, Foam Sclerotherapy, Endovascular Laser, and Radiofrequency Closure. Dermatol Clin. 2005;23:443–5.
3. Subramonia S, Lees TA. The treatment of varicose veins. Ann R Coll Surg Engl. 2007;89:96–100.
4. Bergan JJ et al. Surgical and endovascular treatment of lower extremity venous insufficiency. J Vasc Interv Radiol. 2002;13:563–8.
5. Min R et al. Endovenous laser treatment of the incompetent great saphenous vein. J Vasc Interv Radiol. 2001;12:1167–71.
6. Khilnani NM, Grassi CJ, Kundu S, D'Agostino HR, et al. Multi-society consensus quality improvement guidelines for the treatment of lower-extremity superficial venous insufficiency with endovenous thermal ablation from the Society of Interventional Radiology, Cardiovascular Interventional Radiological Society of Europe, American College of Phlebology, and Canadian Interventional Radiology Association. J Vasc Interv Radiol. 2010;21(1):14–31.

7. Min RJ, Khilnani NM, Golia P. Duplex ultrasound evaluation of lower extremity venous insufficiency. J Vasc Interv Radiol. 2003;14(10):1233–41.
8. Merchant RF, Pichot O. Long term outcomes of endovenous radiofrequency obliteration of saphenous reflux as a treatment for superficial venous insufficiency. J Vasc Surg. 2005;42(3):502–9. discussion 509.
9. Rigby KA, Palfreyman SJ, Beverley C, Michaels JA. Surgery versus sclerotherapy for the treatment of varicose veins. Cochrane Database Syst Rev. 2004;Oct 18;(4): CD004980.
10. Lurie F et al. Prospective randomized study of endovenous radiofrequency obliteration (closure procedure) versus ligation and stripping in a selected patient population (EVOLVeS Study). J Vasc Surg. 2003;38:207–14.
11. Lurie F et al. Prospective randomised study of endovenous radiofrequency obliteration (closure) versus ligation and vein stripping (EVOLVeS): two-year follow-up. Eur J Vasc Endovasc Surg. 2005;29:67–73.
12. Puggioni A, Karla M. Endovenous laser therapy and radiofrequency ablation of the great saphenous vein: analysis of early efficacy and complications. J Vasc Surg. 2005;42(3): 488–93.
13. Huang Y, Jiang M. Endovenous laser treatment combined with a surgical strategy for treatment of venous insufficiency in lower extremity: a report of 208 cases. J Vasc Surg. 2005;42(3):494–501. discussion 501.
14. Rasmussen LH et al. Randomized trial comparing endovenous laser ablation of the great saphenous vein with high ligation and stripping in patients with varicose veins: short-term results. J Vasc Surg. 2007;46:308–15.
15. Wollmann J-C. The history of sclerosing foams. Dermatol Surg. 2004;30(5):694–703.
16. Yamaki T, Nozaki M, Iwasaka S. Comparative study of duplex-guided foam sclerotherapy and duplex-guided liquid sclerotherapy for the treatment of superficial venous insufficiency. Dermatol Surg. 2004;30(5):718–22. discussion 722.
17. Zimmet SE. Hyaluronidase in the prevention of sclerotherapy-induced extravasation necrosis. A dose-response study. Dermatol Surg. 1996;22(1):73–6.
18. D'Othee BJ, Faintuch S, Schirmang T, Lang EV. Endovenous laser ablation of the saphenous veins: bilateral versus unilateral single-session procedures. J Vasc Interv Radiol. 2008;19(2):211–5.
19. Chong PFS, Kumar R, Kushwaha R, Sweeney A, Chaloner EJ. Technical tip: cold saline infiltration instead of local anaesthetic in endovenous laser treatment. Phlebology. 2006;21:88–9.
20. Scultetus AH, Villavicencio JL, Kao TC, et al. Microthrombectomy reduces postsclerotherapy pigmentation: multicenter randomized trial. J Vasc Surg. 2003;38(5):896–903.
21. Rigby KA, Palfreyman SJ, Beverley C, Michaels JA. Surgery versus sclerotherapy for the treatment of varicose veins. Cochrane Database Syst Rev. 2004;18(4):CD004980.
22. Min RJ et al. Endovenous laser treatment of saphenous vein reflux: long-term results. J Vasc Interv Radiol. 2003;14:991–6.

Index

E.A. Ignacio and A.C. Venbrux (eds.), *Women's Health in Interventional Radiology*,
DOI 10.1007/978-1-4419-5876-1, © Springer Science+Business Media, LLC 2012

Printed in the United States
By Bookmasters